Norbert Rietbrock
Barry G. Woodcock (Eds.)

Clinical Pharmacology in the Aged

Klinische Pharmakologie im Alter

N. Rietbrock and B. G. Woodcock (Eds.)

Methods in Clinical Pharmacology

Proceedings Series of the Annual International Symposia held in Frankfurt

Number 1
Methods in Clinical Pharmacology,
co-edited by G. Neuhaus. 1980

Number 2
Progress in Protein Binding,
volume assisted by A. Laßmann. 1981

Number 3
Theophylline and other Methylxanthines,
co-edited by A. H. Staib. 1982

Number 4
Color Vision in Clinical Pharmacology. 1983

Number 5
Balanced Alpha/Beta Blockade of Adrenoceptors.
A Rational Therapeutic Concept in the Treatment
of Hypertension and Coronary Heart Disease. 1984

Number 6
Clinical Pharmacology in the Aged. 1985

Norbert Rietbrock, Barry G. Woodcock (Eds.)

Methods in Clinical Pharmacology
Number 6

Clinical Pharmacology in the Aged

Proceedings of the 6th International Symposium on Methods in Clinical Pharmacology Frankfurt 1985

Klinische Pharmakologie im Alter

Vorträge des 6. Internationalen Symposiums „Methods in Clinical Pharmacology" Frankfurt 1985

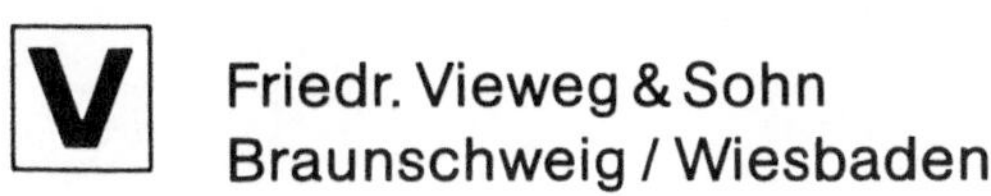

Friedr. Vieweg & Sohn
Braunschweig / Wiesbaden

The Editors

Norbert Rietbrock is Professor of Clinical Pharmacology, *Barry G. Woodcock*
is Senior Lecturer in Clinical Pharmacology, University Clinic,
Frankfurt am Main, Federal Republic of Germany

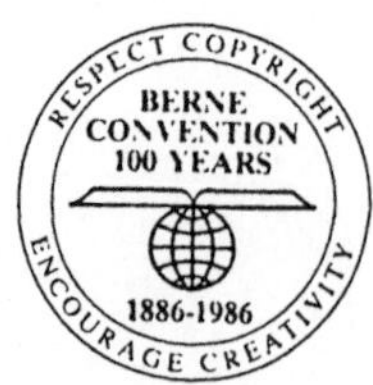

Set by Vieweg, Braunschweig
Produced by Lengericher Handelsdruckerei, Lengerich

ISBN 978-3-528-07935-2   ISBN 978-3-322-89728-2 (eBook)
DOI 10.1007/978-3-322-89728-2

"It is certainly too early to talk about 'gerontopharmacology' as an independent discipline ... nevertheless, ... the principles of pharmacology have to be modified when applied to the elderly."

M. Bergener

Contents / Inhaltsverzeichnis

Einführung

Auf der Erde leben ca. 4,4 Milliarden Menschen. Davon sind 600 Millionen älter als 60 Jahre. Ältere Frauen mit einer größeren Krankheitsanfälligkeit als Männer werden mehr gesundheitlicher und sozialer Betreuung bedürfen. Ältere Menschen suchen häufiger den Arzt auf als jüngere. Dieses zeigt sich in einem überproportional hohen Anteil an Rentnern in den allgemeinen und internistischen Praxen.

Ältere Menschen haben einen durchschnittlich hohen Arzneimittelverbrauch. Aus Berichten verschiedener europäischer Länder geht hervor, daß für die über 60jährigen 30 bis 40% der Aufwendungen auf Arzneimittel entfallen. 75% über 75 Jahre nehmen sogar regelmäßig Arzneimittel ein, 2/3 davon nehmen 2 bis 3 Medikamente täglich, die Hälfte 4 bis 6 Medikamente. Fast 40% der Frauen über 75 Jahre konsumieren regelmäßig psychotrope Mittel. Ein Teil der Aufwendungen ist bei über 65jährigen Patienten überproportional hoch, nämlich bei den Herz-Kreislauferkrankungen, beim Bluthochdruck, bei Stoffwechselerkrankungen wie Diabetes und Befindlichkeitsstörungen. Physiologische Alterung und Polymorbidität führen bei älteren Menschen zwangsläufig, zumindest in der Anfangsphase der Behandlung, zu einer Polypragmasie in der Pharmakotherapie. Daraus erwächst wiederum die Gefahr, daß bei Einnahme mehrerer Medikamente Nebenwirkungen und Interaktionen gehäuft auftreten. Auch die Zahl der Todesfälle durch Nebenwirkungen von Arzneimitteln scheinen mit dem Alter anzuwachsen. Unter 10 000 Obduktionen der Heidelberger und Darmstädter pathologischen Institute wurden morphologische Manifestationen von Arzneimittelschäden in 2,6% der Fälle nachgewiesen. Von 257 Fällen waren 34,6% mit Arzneimittelschäden die Haupttodesursache. In 17,5% stellten sie einen wesentlichen Befund dar, während sie in 26,8% als Nebenbefunde auftraten. In 20,6% der Fälle war die Schädigung durch ein Arzneimittel nicht vom Grundleiden zu trennen (Platt). Diese Zahlen sind für den Kenner der Materie alarmierend, auch angesichts der unbekannten Dunkelziffer von Todesfällen durch Arzneimittel bei alten Menschen. Offenbar wird der Verschreibung von Arzneimitteln mit geringer therapeutischer Breite an betagte Personen zu wenig Aufmerksamkeit geschenkt. Unbekannt ist, warum sich die konservative restriktive Grundeinstellung des Kinderarztes, sich auf wenige langerprobte Medikamente zu beschränken, ferner auf das Alter, das Körpergewicht oder auf den Funktionszustand der Organe zu achten, noch immer bei Verordnung im höheren Lebensalter vermißt wird. Gerade in dieser Lebensphase finden gravierende Veränderungen im Wasserhaushalt, Verschiebungen innerhalb der Flüssigkeitsräume, Abnahme der Muskelmasse, Zunahme des Fettgewebes u. a. statt.

Nicht alle Arzneimittelwirkungen sind beim älteren Menschen erkennbar und nicht alle unerwarteten Wirkungen sind dramatisch. Es gilt das Unvernünftige zu unterlassen aber das, was therapeutisch vernünftig ist, zu tun.

Einige von Ihnen kennen vielleicht das Märchen der Brüder Grimm, beide geboren in Hanau unweit von Frankfurt, Jakob der ältere 1785 und Wilhelm der jüngere 1786.

Danach wurde dem Menschen vom Schöpfer ursprünglich 30 Lebensjahre zugestanden. Mit dieser knapp bemessenen Lebensspanne war der Mensch aber unzufrieden, und so nahm der Herrgott dem Esel, dem Hund und dem Affen einige Jahre ab und gab sie dem Menschen. Demgemäß hat nun der Mensch die ersten 30 Jahre seines Lebens wirklich zueigen. Die nächsten 18 Jahre muß er sich placken wie ein Esel. Zwischen dem 48. und 60. Lebensjahr liegt er dann in der Ecke, knurrend und zahnlos wie ein alter Hund, und wenn es hochkommt, sind ihm noch 10 weitere Lebensjahre beschieden, in denen er närrisch wird wie ein Affe.

Das Alter beschrieben als Abfall, als Verlust, als Defizit von Fähigkeiten und Leistungen, als Einschränkung des Verhaltensradius.

Ein ähnliches Bild vom alternden Menschen zeichnet Jean Paul in „Die wunderbare Gesellschaft", wenn er sagt: „Bettet doch alte Menschen weich und warm und lasset sie recht genießen, denn weiter vermögen sie nichts mehr; und bescheret ihnen gerade im Lebens-Dezember und in ihren längsten Nächten Weihnachtsfeiertage und Christbäume; sie sind ja auch Kinder, ja Zurückwachsende."

Vernünftig ist daher — und ich greife den unterbrochenen Gedanken wieder auf — die Einstellung der Gesellschaft zum alten Menschen zu verbessern.

Paul Morawitz hat 1932 bei Eröffnung des Wiesbadener Internisten Kongresses, weit seiner Zeit voraus, gesagt: „Es wird die Zeit kommen und vielleicht schneller als wir denken, in der es nicht mehr genügen wird, pathologisch — anatomische Diagnosen zu stellen, sondern in der zur Beurteilung des Krankheitsbildes auch Berücksichtigung der individuellen körperlichen und seelischen Struktur verlangt werden wird. Es wird nicht mehr allein gefragt: „Was hat dieser Patient für eine Krankheit?" — sondern auch: „Was ist das für ein Mensch, wie ist er beschaffen?" Der ältere Mensch steht in der Tat in einem Spannungsfeld, wo gesundmachende und krankmachende Kräfte auf ihn einwirken. Zwar hat er Erfahrungen über sich selbst und seine Umwelt gesammelt. Er hat stärker und intensiver über die Vergänglichkeit und Nichtigkeit aller menschlichen Aktivitäten nachgedacht. Existentielle Veränderungen, Anpassung an eine neue Umwelt, Verlust des familiären Milieus, Verstecktwerden in Altersheimen haben aber nachteilige und oft krankmachende Folgen. Dieses sollte uns allen bewußt sein."

Zu einer vernünftigen sozialen Betreuung gehört auch eine vernünftige medikamentöse Therapie. Ihr gegenüber steht die Unvernunft einer Übermedikamentierung der alten Menschen diametral. Wir finden gerade bei der Behandlung der alten Menschen Übermedikation in Form der gedankenlosen ärztlichen Polypragmasie u.a. in der sinnlosen Verschreibung von unwirksamen Geriatrika, in der Verschreibung von beliebig vielen Arzneimitteln, überflüssiger Kombinationspräparate und in der Verordnung von Medikamenten bei „non-diseases". Erfahrungsmedizin ohne den Versuch eines Wirksamkeitsnachweises ist spekulative Medizin. Bewahren wir unsere älteren Mitbürger vor diesen Spekulationen.

Ich möchte mich bei allen Mitarbeitern der Abteilung für die Mitwirkung bei der Ausrichtung des Symposiums bedanken. Ebenso bedanke ich mich bei den Damen und Herren der Firma Merck für ihre finanzielle Unterstützung.

May I thank you all for coming to Frankfurt. We are most happy to welcome our friends from the United States, Ireland, Scotland, England and Wales.

Norbert Rietbrock

I The Aging Phenomenon and Its Impact on Therapeutics and Prescribing

Perspectives in Biogerontology

L. Hayflick
Center for Gerontological Studies, University of Florida, 3357 Turlington Hall, Gainesville, Florida 32611, USA

Summary

After reaching sexual maturity, individual members of a species accumulate physiological decrements that lead to an increase in their likelihood of dying. This decline in function is called aging. For man, the likelihood of dying doubles every seven years beyond the age of 30.

The triumphs of modern medicine have not lengthened the human lifespan. Medical successes merely have permitted more people to reach what appears to be a fixed upper age limit. Life expectation has increased but life span has not. In many developed countries, one can now reasonably expect to become old, which is a very new phenomenon.

If the two leading causes of death in developed countries were to be eliminated (cardiovascular diseases and cancer), about 14 years of additional life expectation would occur for all age groups. Resolving all other causes of death would add an additional 2 years of life expectation. Thus if all causes of premature death were to be eliminated, all humans would live to be about 100 years of age. They would then die as the result of normal losses in physiological function which previously increased their vulnerability to an earlier death caused by disease or accidents. The diseases of old age are simply superimposed on the normal physiological decrements that occur after sexual maturation.

Studies on isolated human cells grown in laboratory cultures indicate that normal cells have a limited capacity to divide and to function. They have a chronometer that limits their replicative and functional capacity. Cells grown in culture from older donors have a reduced capacity to divide and function when compared to cells grown from younger donors. Before cells die in culture they reveal several hundred changes, many of which are similar to those changes that occur in the intact older human.

Current evidence leads to the belief that age changes are substantially due to changes that occur in the genetic machinery of individual cells. The changes apparently are induced by the same genetic program that operates throughout the life of the individual.

Introduction

Of all the conflicting views on the causes of biologic aging, few gerontologists disagree with the axiom that after reaching sexual maturity and cessation of growth, animals accumulate physiologic decrements that lead to an increase in their likelihood of dying. In fact, for humans, the data, first analyzed by the English actuary Gompertz in 1825, reveal that the force of mortality doubles every 7 years after the age of 30. That is, after maturity, the rate and probability of dying are exponential with increasing age. A variety of human physiologic functions, although subject to some individual variation, show a slow, nearly linear decline from 30 years of age. The rate constants for this linear loss seem to occur at about 0.8 to 0.9 percent loss per year of the functional capacity present at the age of 30 (Strehler and Mildvan, 1960).

The common impression that the triumphs of modern medicine have lengthened the human lifespan is not supported by either vital statistics or biologic evidence. The fact is that in the developed countries, the prevention and treatment of ills which occur in the early years has improved, permitting more people to reach what appears to be an immutable, upper age limit. Thus life expectation has increased, but the human lifespan has remained virtually unchanged for several hundred thousand years.

Medical achievements have simply allowed more people to reach the limit of that fixed lifespan. Deaths in the early years are becoming increasingly less frequent in the developed countries, resulting in life tables that are simply becoming more rectangular. In many privileged countries, one can now expect to become reasonably old, which is a relatively new phenomenon.

Effects of the Resolution of Diseases

If cardiovascular diseases, which are the leading cause of death in the United States, are prevented, approximately 12 years of additional life can be expected (Table I). If the second greatest cause of death — cancer — is eliminated, about 2 years of additional

Table I: Gain in expectation of life at birth and at age 65 due to elimination of various causes of death. 1969—71

Cause of Death	Gain (year) in Expectation of Life if Cause was Eliminated	
	At birth	At age of 65
Major cardiovascular-renal diseases	11.8	11.4
Diseases of the heart	5.9	5.1
Cerebrovascular diseases	1.2	1.2
Malignant neoplasms*	2.5	1.4
Motor vehicle accidents	0.7	0.1
All accidents excluding motor vehicles	0.6	0.1
Influenza and pneumonia	0.5	0.2
Diabetes mellitus	0.2	0.2
Infectious and parasitic diseases	0.2	0.1
Tuberculosis	Less than 0.05	

* Including neoplasms of lymphatic and hematopoietic tissues.

Source: U.S. Public Health Service, National Center for Health Statistics, "U.S. Life Tables by Causes of Death: 1969—71," by T.N.E. Greville, "U.S. Decennial Life Tables for 1969—71," Vol. 1, No. 5, 1976.

life expectation will result. The net increase in life expectancy at birth achieved in the United States from 1900 to 1985 was about 25 years. This increase resulted from the decrease in the large number of deaths that occurred before the age of 65. However, the gain in life expectancy at 65 and 75 years of age from 1900 to 1969 was, respectively, only 2.9 and 2.2 years.

What would be the effect on human longevity and the human lifespan in a world in which all causes of death resulting from disease and accidents were totally eliminated (Table I)? The effect on human longevity would be to realize the ultimate rectangular curve in which citizens would live out their lives free of the fear of premature death, but with the certain knowledge that their normal physiologic decrements would result in death on about their 100th birthday.

These concepts have forced gerontologists to the conclusion that the disease-oriented approach to medical research might increase life expectation but will have little impact on increasing the human lifespan. If such an increase is desirable (and there is considerable doubt that it is), one must first separate the disease-related causes of death from the age-dependent normal physiologic decrements that give rise to the manifestations of old age. The diseases of old age are simply superimposed on these normal physiologic decrements but must be separately regarded to consider ways of increasing the human lifespan. Although age-associated physiologic decrements surely increase vulnerability to disease, the fundamental causes of death are not diseases, (or many kinds of accidents) but the physiologic decrements that make their occurrence more likely.

Biomedical research has directed its efforts almost exclusively on the disease-associated causes of death. Scant attention has been paid to the underlying causes of biologic aging that are not disease-associated, but which, in clocklike fashion, dictate for each species a specific maximum lifespan. To be sure, the physiologic decrements that occur in advancing years increase vulnerability to disease, but unless more attention is paid to the fundamental non-disease-related biologic causes of aging, the fate of each person will be death on about his or her 100th birthday.

Prospects for Increasing Human Longevity

As stated, there are two ways in which the efforts of biomedical research can be expected to extend human longevity. The first is to reduce or eliminate the major causes of death. For most developed countries, this would mean eliminating cardiovascular diseases and cancer. In the developing countries, life expectancy can be extended by the simple expedient of motivating the political and economic infrastructure to provide citizens with the necessary food, hygienic conditions, and medical care that are commonplace in developed countries. The results of reducing the role of minor diseases in developed countries will be minimal. For example, in the United States, if tuberculosis were completely eliminated, the gain in life expectation at birth would be less than 0.05 year (Table I). Thus it could be argued that if an increase in life expectation becomes the main goal of biomedical research in the developed countries, research should be directed toward the elimination of the two major causes of death. This position, although less than humane and not likely to attract many adherents, is nonetheless the most logical conclusion to be drawn from life-table studies and the projections dealt with in Table I.

The second way in which biomedical research can deal with human longevity is to address itself specifically to the underlying nondisease-related fundamental causes of age changes. These are not diseases but are the basic biological changes that result in the physiological decrements characteristic of normal aging. On these changes is superimposed an increasing vulnerability to disease. Such an approach, then, does not directly concern itself with efforts to increase human life expectation but rather to extend what appears to be a fixed lifespan.

As a measure of the current effort put forth toward these two approaches, funds spent in the United States on cardiovascular disease and cancer research are about twenty times greater than the funds spent in biogerontology. It is also probable that the number of researchers, and consequently the amount of effort, in both these areas also differs by twenty-fold. Consequently, the likelihood that any significant increase in human longevity will occur in the next 15 years depends on (1) significantly better cure rates for cardiovascular diseases or cancer or both, and (2) significant advances in our understanding and ability to manipulate the biological clocks that have set a maximum lifespan for each of us.

Demographic Projections

That the proportion of persons in developed countries over the age of 65 has been steadily increasing is well known. In the last 100 years, their proportion of the total population in the United States has increased from 3.4 to 11.6 percent.

Within 50 years, those over 65 are expected to number nearly 40 million in the United States. This prediction does not take into account any major resolution within 50 years of the two leading causes of death — cardiovascular disease and cancer. If some significant cure rate were to occur, however, the United States might have as many persons over 65 as under 15 in the year 2025.

Aging at the Cellular Level

The notion that aging occurs in animals that reach a fixed size after maturity is beyond dispute. But is the inevitability of the aging and death of individual cells composing that organism predetermined? A superficial consideration of this thought may provoke some incredulity since it is intuitively obvious that a dead or aging organism must consist of dead or aging cells. Nevertheless, whatever causes age changes and death in the whole organism undoubtedly does not produce similar changes, and at the same rate, in each cell composing that organism. If the rates of aging vary among organs, tissues, and their constituent cells, then the root causes of aging may occur as a consequence of decrements in some few cell types where the rate is fastest and the effects greatest. Let us explore the notion that normal somatic cells are predestined to undergo irreversible functional decrements that lead to aging in the whole organism.

There are at least two ways in which this question has been put to the test. First, vertebrate cells have been serially cultured in laboratory glassware, and second, similar cells, containing specific markers allowing them to be distinguished from host cells, have been serially transplanted in isogenic laboratory animals. The goals of such studies, as they pertain to the science of gerontology, have been directed toward answering this fundamental question: Can vertebrate cells, functioning and replicating under ideal conditions, escape from the inevitability of aging and death that is universally characteristic of the whole animals from which they were derived?

8

In respect to studies undertaken in cell culture, one investigation stands out as the classic response to this intriguing question. In the early part of this century, Alexis Carrel, a noted cell culturist, described experiments purporting to show that the fibroblasts derived from chick heart tissue could be cultured seriatim indefinitely. The culture was voluntarily terminated after 34 years. This experiment is important to gerontologists because it implied that if cells released from in vivo control could divide and function normally for a period in excess of the lifespan of a species, then either the types of cells cultured play no role in the aging phenomenon or aging is the result of changes occurring at the supracellular level. That is, aging would be the result of decrements that occur only in organized tissue or whole organs as a result of the physiologic interactions between those organized cell hierarchies. The inference would be that aging per se is not the result of events occurring at the cell level.

In the years that followed Carrel's observations, support for his experimental results seemed to be forthcoming from the many laboratories in which it was observed that cultured cell populations, derived from many tissues of a variety of animal species and from humans, had the striking ability to replicate apparently indefinitely. These cell populations number in the hundreds and are best known by the prototype cell lines HeLa (derived from a human cervical carcinoma in 1952) and L cells (derived from mouse mesenchyme in 1943). They continue to flourish even to this day in cell-culture laboratories throughout the world. They arise by some unknown spontaneous process, or they can be purposely provoked by the introduction of chemical carcinogens or certain oncogenic viruses into cultures of normal cells. Nevertheless, what seemed to be incontrovertible evidence for the potential immortality of vertebrate cells soon fell to new insights and a preponderance of opposing evidence.

Aging Under Glass

Of central importance to the question is whether the cell populations studied in vitro are composed of normal or abnormal cells. Clearly the aging of animals occurs in normal cell populations. If we are to equate the behavior of normal cells in vivo with that of similar cells in vitro, then the latter must be shown to be normal as well. For this reason the "immortal" cell lines described earlier, of which the HeLa and L cell populations are prototypes, must be excluded from consideration because they are composed of cells that are abnormal in one or more important properties. For example, all immortal cell lines vary in their chromosomal constitution; they do not reveal either the exact number or the precise morphology of chromosomes characteristic of the cells composing the tissue of origin. The widespread use of these cells lines for a variety of research purposes in laboratories throughout the world is subject to the criticism that in most cases they are not characteristic of any cell type found in human or animal tissue. Much experimental data generated from the use of such cell populations cannot be extrapolated to apply to cells that characterize the animal species from which they originally descended. Consequently, the use of cell lines is questionable because such cells undoubtedly represent laboratory artifacts whose behavior may be unrelated to cells found in vivo.

This fundamental flaw in interpreting normal cell behavior in vitro can, in fact, be circumvented. Cell populations entirely typical of normal cells found in vivo can be cultured, and with respect to gerontologic inquiry, the findings are profoundly different from the behavior of abnormal cell lines.

Twenty-five years ago, Paul Moorhead and I found that cultured normal human embryonic fibroblasts underwent a finite number of serial subcultivations or population doublings and then they died (Hayflick and Moorhead, 1961). We demonstrated that when such cells were grown under the most favorable conditions, death was inevitable after about 50 population doublings (the Phase III Phenomenon). We also showed that the death of the normal cells was not due to some trivial explanation involving medium components or cultural conditions, but that the death of cultured normal cells was an inherent property of the cells themselves. That observation has now been confirmed in hundreds of laboratories in which variations in medium components and cultural conditions have been as numerous as the laboratories themselves (Hayflick and Moorhead, 1961 and Hayflick, 1965).

Since normal diploid cell strains have a limited doubling potential in vitro, studies on any single strain would be severely curtailed were it not possible to preserve these cells at subzero temperatures for apparently indefinite periods of time. The reconstitution of frozen human fetal diploid cell strains has revealed that regardless of the doubling level reached by the population at the time it is preserved, the total number of doublings that can be expected is about 50 when those made before and after preservation are combined. Storage of human diploid cell strains merely arrests the cells at a particular population doubling level but does not influence the total number of expected doublings (Hayflick and Moorhead, 1961 and Hayflick, 1965).

We have reconstituted about 130 ampules of our human fetal diploid cell strain WI-38, which was placed in liquid nitrogen storage 24 years ago. All have yielded cell populations that have undergone 50 ± 10 cumulative population doublings. This represents the longest period of time that viable normal human cells have been arrested at subzero temperatures.

Since normal human embryo fibroblasts are able to undergo only a fixed number of reproductive cycles in vitro, we postulated that this observation might be interpreted as aging at the cell level. Although we and others were skeptical of this interpretation at first, subsequent experimental data have tended to support the validity of this notion. I have named the burgeoning field of cellular aging, cytogerontology. However, before considering the newer developments in this fields, it is necessary to reconsider Carrel's experiment, in which a presumptive normal chicken cell population was cultured for 34 years and then voluntarily terminated. The cells cultured by Carrel are presumed to have been normal. In the years following Carrel's observation, and even in very recent times when more sophisticated cell-culture techniques have been used, there has been only one report of an abnormal, chick fibroblast culture propagated serially for more than 1 year (Ogura, Fujiwara and Namba, 1984). Thus there is serious doubt that the original interpretation of Carrel's work can be accepted unless one assumes that his alleged immortal cell population was, in fact, an abnormal cell line. In that case it has no bearing on cell aging. I have proposed one explanation for Carrel's findings that was subsequently supported by personal communications from one of his laboratory technicians. The method of preparation of chick embryo extract, used as a source of nutrients for his cultures and prepared daily under conditions of low-speed centrifugation, allowed for the survival and introduction of new, viable fibroblasts into the so-called immortal culture at each feeding (Hayflick, 1970 and Hayflick, 1972). Although Carrel may have been unaware of this, others believe otherwise (Witkowski, 1985).

Donor Age Versus Cell Doubling Potential

Because cultured normal human cells derived from embryonic tissue have a finite proliferative capacity of about 50 population doublings and because this may represent cellular aging, it is important to determine the proliferative capacity of normal cells derived from human adults of varying ages. Our first report of such studies did indeed show a diminished proliferative capacity for cultured normal human adult fibroblasts in which 14 to 29 doublings occurred in cells derived from 8 adult donors (Hayflick, 1965). This compared with a range of 35 to 63 doublings found in cells cultured from 13 human embryos.

Subsequent to these studies a report by Martin, Sprague and Epstein, 1970, not only confirmed the principle we observed but extended it significantly. These investigators cultured fibroblasts derived from biopsies taken from the upper arm of human donors ranging from fetal to 90 years of age. They found the regression coefficient, from the first to the ninth decade, to be -0.20 population doublings per year of life with a standard deviation of 0.05 and a correlation coefficient of -0.50.

In the past 14 years, several additional studies on human tissues have been reported. LeGuilly, Simon, Lenoir and Bourel, 1973 used human liver tissue, Schneider and Mitsui, 1976; Goldstein, Moerman, Soeldner, Gleason and Barnett, 1978; and Vracko and Mc-Farland, 1980 studied fibroblasts from skin biopsies, Bierman, 1978 examined arterial smooth-muscle cells, Tassin, Malaise and Courtois, 1979 used lens cells and Walford, Jarwaid and Naeim, 1981 and Walford, 1982 used T-lymphocytes. All of these studies tend to support our original contention that the number of population doublings achievable by cultured normal human cells is inversely proportional to donor age (Hayflick, 1965). Nevertheless, these findings must be tempered with observations that the relationship may be clouded when different tissue sites are compared (Schneider, Mitsui, Aw and Schorr, 1977) or where the physiologic state of the donor is abnormal. For example, strains derived from diabetics have been found to undergo fewer doublings in vitro than their normal, age-matched counterparts (Goldstein, Moerman, Soeldner, Gleason and Barnett, 1978).

Direct Proportionality Between Maximum Species Life Span and Population Doubling Potential

Several years ago I suggested that the population doubling potential of cultured fibroblasts from several animal species revealed a surprisingly good direct correlation with maximum species lifespan (Hayflick, 1976). In the years that followed several other reports have appeared that have substantiated this idea, especially that of Rohme, 1981. One report in which several marsupial species were studied does not support this finding, however, the authors did not determine population doublings by conventional means nor is the maximum lifespans of the species they studied known (Stanley, Pye, and MacGregor, 1975). Fig. 1 shows the direct proportionality between different species maximum life spans and the population doubling potential of their cultured fibroblasts. Embryonic fibroblasts were used in the ten species studied except that of the Galapagos tortoise where cells from a juvenile were used.

If this relationship is extended and confirmed it suggests the presence of a chronometer or pacemaker within all normal cells that is characteristic for each species and that dictates maximum cell doubling or functional capacity with an apparent evolutionary

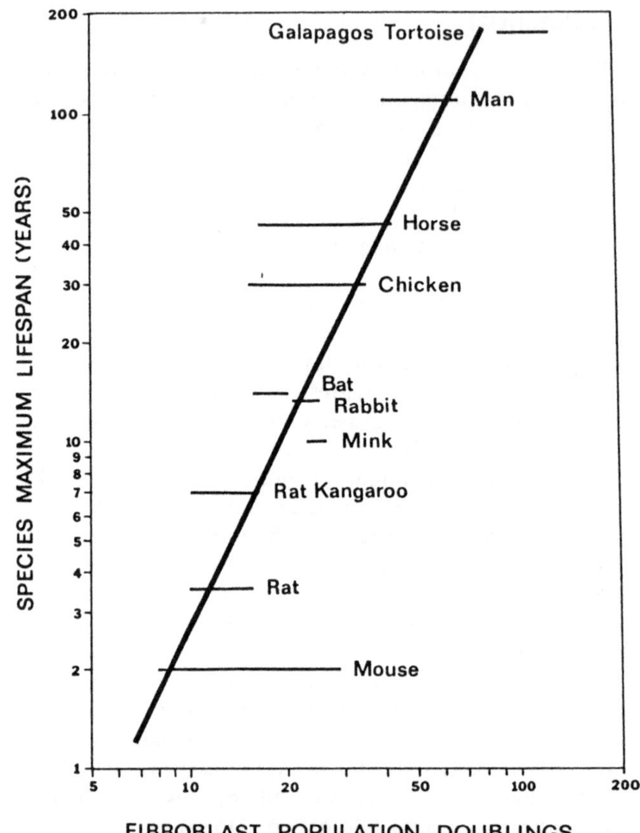

Fig. 1
Range of population doublings found for cultured normal fibroblasts derived from the embroynic tissue of several vertebrate species. Galapagos tortoise tissue was obtained from a juvenile animal.

basis. The postulated chronometer may or may not be the same one that we postulate controls the inverse relationship between donor age and population doubling potential.

Progeria and Werner's Syndrome

Progeria (Hutchinson-Guilford syndrome) is a human condition leading to a severe deceleration of growth in patients as young as 9 years of age (Reichel, Garcia-Bunuel, and Dilallo, 1971). A very rare disease, it is thought by many to represent a model for precocious aging in which individuals, at the end of the first decade of life, manifest the physical signs of aging typical of their normal counterparts in the seventh decade of life. Werner's syndrome is similar to progeria in many ways, although its salient manifestations occur in later years. The full clinical picture shows early graying and loss of hair, short stature, juvenile cataracts, proneness to diabetes, atherosclerosis and calcification of the blood vessels, osteoporosis, and high incidence of malignancy (Epstein, Martin, Schultz and Motulsky, 1966).

If Werner's syndrome and progeria are examples of accelerated aging, when does senescence of cultured fibroblasts taken from these patients occur? From 2 to 10 doublings were found to occur, whereas normal values would be between 20 and 40 (Martin, Sprague and Epstein, 1970; Goldstein, 1969; Goldstein, 1971). Others have reported decreased mitotic activity, DNA synthesis, and cloning efficiency of cultured progeria cells (Danes, 1971; Nienhaus, DeJong, and Tenkate, 1971).

The Finite Lifetime of Normal Cells in Vivo

If the concept of the finite lifetime or senescence of normal cells replicating in vitro is related to aging in the whole animal, then it is important to know whether normal cells, given the opportunity, can proliferate indefinitely in vivo.

If all the multitude of animal cell types were continually renewed, without loss of function or capacity for self-renewal, we would expect that the organs composed of such cells would function normally indefinitely and that their host would live forever. Unhappily, however, renewal cell populations do not occur in most tissues, and when they do, a proliferative finitude is often manifest. Although this important question has been discussed previously, much new information has become available in recent years (Hayflick, 1970; Hayflick, 1977; Hayflick, 1980).

It is apparent that animals whose growth stops after sexual maturity have a specific lifespan and then die. The normal somatic cells composing their tissues obviously die as well. The important question then is: Is it possible to circumvent the death of normal animal cells that result from the death of the "host" by transferring marked cells to younger animals seriatim? If such experiments could be devised, then we would have an in vivo counterpart of the in vitro experiments and would predict that normal cells transplanted serially to proper inbred hosts would, like their in vitro counterparts, age. Such experiments would largely rule out those objections to in vitro findings that are based on the artificiality of in vitro cell cultures. The question could be answered by serial orthotopic transplantation of normal somatic tissue to new, young, inbred hosts each time the recipient approaches old age.

Data from seven different laboratories in which mammary tissue (Daniel, deOme, Young, Blair and Faulkin, 1968), skin (Krohn, 1962), and hematopoietic cells (Ford, Micklem, and Gray, 1959; Cudkowicz, Upton, Shearer and Hughes, 1964; Siminovitch, Till and McCulloch, 1964; Harrison, 1973; Harrison, 1975, 1985 and Hellman, Botnick, Hannon and Vigneulle, 1978) were employed indicate that normal cells serially transplanted to inbred hosts do not survive indefinitely. Furthermore, the trauma of transplantation does not appear to influence the results (Krohn, 1962). And finally, in heterochronic transplants, survival time is related to the age of the grafted tissue (Krohn, 1962). It is well known that under similar conditions of tissue transplantation, cancer cell populations can be serially passed indefinitely (Stewart, Snell, Dunham and Schylen, 1959; Daniel, Aidells, Medina and Faulkin, 1975; and Till, McCulloch and Siminovitch, 1964). The implications of this may be that acquisition of potential for unlimited cell division or escape from senescent changes by mammalian cells in vitro or in vivo can only be achieved by somatic cells that have acquired some or all of the properties of cancer cells.

Paradoxically, this leads to the conclusion that in order for mammalian somatic cells to become biologically "immortal", they first must be induced to an abnormal or neoplastic state either in vivo or in vitro, at which time they can be subcultivated or transplanted indefinitely. Krohn, 1962 found some transplants capable of surviving several years beyond the maximum lifespan of the mouse, but they were ultimately lost. It is important to note that long survival time is not equivalent to proliferation time or rounds of division; hence these long-surviving grafts consist of cells having a very slow rate of reproductive turnover. This is analogous to holding cell cultures at room temperature, which also extends calendar time for cell survival but does not result in an increase in population doublings.

A series of experiments has been reported that clearly shows that the birth rate of mouse mammary epithelium declines during in vivo serial transplantation (Daniel, deOme, Young, Blair and Faulkin, 1968; Daniel and Young, 1971; Daniel, 1973). Mouse mammary epithelium was propagated in isogenic female hosts by periodic transplantation of tissue samples into the mammary fat pads from which the host gland was surgically removed. These workers repeatedly observed that unlike cancerous and precancerous mammary tissue, normal mammary epithelium displays a characteristic decline in proliferative capacity with repeated transplantation (Daniel, deOme, Young, Blair and Faulkin, 1968). It also has been found that when transplants that are allowed to proliferate continuously are compared with transplants in which growth is restricted, the decline in cell proliferation is related to number of population doublings undergone rather than to the passage of metabolic time (Daniel and Young, 1971). This represents the first in vivo confirmation of our in vitro data (Hayflick and Moorhead, 1961; Hayflick, 1965). At that time, we suggested that somatic cells have an intrinsic, predetermined capacity for division under the most favorable environmental conditions. Others, (Hay and Strehler, 1967; McHale, Moulton and McHale, 1971) however, have invoked the passage of "metabolic time" as the determinant of in vitro senescence. That metabolic time is not the governing factor, but that population doublings are has been demonstrated beyond doubt (Dell'Orco, Mertens, Kruse, 1974; Harley and Goldstein, 1978). The in vivo finding that population doublings dictate cell senescence and not "metabolic time" (Daniel and Young, 1971) is especially significant because it results from studies on cells grown entirely in situ and thus circumvents arguments leveled at similar data obtained from the alleged "artificial" conditions of in vitro cell culture. These investigators conclude that "the ability of grafts from old donors to proliferate rapidly in young hosts suggests that the lifespan of mammary glands is influenced primarily by the number of cell divisions rather than by the passage of chronological or metabolic time." (Young, Medina, deOme and Daniel, 1971).

The study of single antibody-forming cell clones in vivo has shown that these cells are also capable of only a limited capacity to replicate after serial transfer in vivo (Williamson and Askonas, 1972; Williamson, 1972). Harrison, 1972 and Harrison, 1973 report that when marrow cell transplants from young and old normal donors are made to a genetically anemic recipient mouse strain, the anemia is cured. He further reports that such transplants to anemic mice ultimately expire, exhibiting once again the finitude of normal cell proliferation in vivo (Harrison, 1975).

In connection with findings that bear on the proliferative capacity of cells in vivo as a function of age, several other intriguing reports should be mentioned here. The most informative of such studies are those bearing on the major cell renewal system: the hematopoietic cells of the bone marrow, the epidermis, the lymphatic cells of the thymus, the spleen and lymph nodes, the sperm cells in the seminiferous tubules of the testes, and the epithelial cells lining the small intestine. It has been found, for example, in the latter system in the mouse that cell generation time increases with age, (Lesher, Fry and Kohn, 1961a, 1961b and Thrasher and Greulich, 1965). The increase in generation time, however, is not a linear increase from early youth to extreme old age (Lesher and Sacher, 1968).

Thus we can see a wide variety of examples of in vivo constraints on the proliferative capacity of replicating cell cohorts. It is likely that different proliferative cell systems may display variations on this general theme. Based on our in vitro data, fibroblasts may represent the upper limit of proliferative potential, although one should not exclude a higher limit being placed on such cell renewal systems as hematopoietic cells or skin epithelium, neither of which have been shown to proliferate in vitro for long periods of time and still retain normal characteristics and functional capacities.

Decrements Occurring in Cultured Normal Human Cells

The probability that animals age because one or more important cell populations lose their proliferative capacity is unlikely. It is more probable that, as we have shown, normal cells have a finite capacity for replication and that this finite limit is rarely, if ever, reached by cells in vivo but is, of course, demonstrable in vitro. We would therefore suggest that other functional losses that occur in cells prior to the cessation of division capacity produce physiologic decrements in animals much before their normal cells have reached their maximum proliferative capacity. Indeed, we are now becoming aware of many functional changes that take place in normal human cells grown in vitro and expressed well before they lose their capacity to replicate (Hayflick, 1980). Over 125 functional changes occur in cultured normal human cells as they age. These changes occur in such things as DNA, RNA, enzymes, cell cycle, karyology, lipids, carbohydrates, morphology, and protein synthesis. It is more likely that these changes, which herald the approaching loss of division capacity, play the central role in the expression of aging and result in the death of the individual animal well before its cells fail to divide (Hayflick, 1976).

To be sure, those several classes of cells which are incapable of division in mature animals, such as neurons and muscle cells, may play a greater role in the expression of age changes than those cell classes in which division commonly occurs. It is important, therefore, to indicate that the cessation of mitotic activity is only one functional decrement whose genetic basis may be similar to those functional decrements known to occur in nondividing cells. It is suggested, therefore, that the same kind of gene action resulting in physiologic decrements in aging nondividing cells also occurs in aging cells that can divide. It is not our contention, therefore, that age changes result necessarily from losses in cell-division capacity, but simply in loss of function in any class of cells. That function might be measured as reduced division capacity or any number of the myriad functional decrements characteristic of aging cells. The genetic changes leading to these decrements are postulated to be the common denominator, so that the measurement of loss of population doubling potential in vitro may have the same basis as the loss of other cell functions characteristic of nondividing cells. It follows, therefore, that an understanding of the mechanism by which cultured normal cells lose their capacity to replicate could provide insights into the causes of decrements in other functional properties that are characteristic of such nondividing cells as neurons. These decrements may be even more direct causes of biologic aging.

Dedication

This paper is dedicated to the memory of Dr. Henry S. Kaplan, Professor of Radiology, Stanford University School of Medicine; scholar, physician, teacher, friend and champion of just causes.

References

Bierman, E. L.: The effect of donor age on the in vitro lifespan of cultured human arterial smooth-muscle cells. In Vitro **14**, 951–955 (1978).

Cudkowicz, G., Upton, A. C., Shearer, G. M., Hughes, W. L.: Lymphocyte content and proliferative capacity of serially transplanted mouse bone marrow. Nature **201**, 165–167 (1964).

Danes, B. S.: Progeria: A cell culture study on aging. J. Clin. Invest. **50**, 2000–2003 (1971).

Daniel, C. W., deOme, K. B., Young, J. T., Blair, P. B., Faulkin, L. J., Jr.: The in vivo lifespan of normal and preneoplastic mouse mammary glands: A serial transplantation study. Proc. Nat. Acad. Sci. U.S.A. **61**, 53–60 (1968).

Daniel, C. W., Young, L. J. T.: Influence of cell division on an aging process. Exp. Cell Res. **65**, 27–32 (1971).

Daniel, C. W.: Finite growth span of mouse mammary gland serially propagated in vivo. Experientia (Basel) **29**, 1422–1424 (1973).

Daniel, C. W., Aidells, B. D., Medina, B., Faulkin, L. J., Jr.: Unlimited division potential of precancerous mouse mammary cells after spontaneous or carcinogen-induced transformation. Fed. Proc. **34**, 64–67 (1975).

Dell'Orco, R. T., Mertens, J. G., Kruse, P. F., Jr.: Doubling potential, calendar time, and donor age of human diploid cells in culture. Exp. Cell Res. **84**, 363–366 (1974).

Epstein, C. J., Martin, G. M., Schultz, A. L., Motulsky, A. G.: Werner's syndrome: A review of its symptomatology, natural history, pathologic features, genetics and relationship to the natural aging process. Medicine (Baltimore) **45**, 177–221 (1966).

Ford, C. E., Micklem, H. S., Gray, S. M: Evidence of selective proliferation of reticular cell-clones in heavily irradiated mice. Br. J. Radiol. **32**, 280 (1959).

Goldstein, S.: Lifespan of cultured cells in progeria. Lancet **1**, 424 (1969).

Goldstein, S.: The biology of aging. N. Engl. J. Med. **285**, 1120–1129 (1971).

Goldstein, S., Moerman, E. J., Soeldner, J. S., Gleason, R. E., Barnett, D. M.: Chronologic and physiologic age effect replicative lifespan of fibroblasts from diabetics, prediabetics, and normal donors. Science **199**, 781–782 (1978).

Harley, C. B., Goldstein, S.: Cultured human fibroblasts: Distribution of cell generations and a critical limit. J. Cell Physiol. **97**, 509–516 (1978).

Harrison, D. E.: Normal function of transplanted mouse erythrocyte precursors for 21 months beyond donor lifespans. Nature New Biol. **237**, 220–222 (1972).

Harrison, D. E.: Normal Production of erythrocytes by mouse marrow continuous for 73 months. Proc. Nat. Acad. Sci. U.S.A. **70**, 3184–3188 (1973).

Harrison, D. E.: Normal function of transplanted marrow cell lines from aged mice. J. Gerontol. **30**, 279–285 (1975).

Harrison, D. E.: Cell and tissue transplantation: a means of studying the aging process. In: C. Finch and E. Schneider (Eds.) Handbook of the Biology of Aging. (pp. 322–356). New York, Van Nostrand Reinhold Co. (1977).

Hay, R. J., Strehler, B. L.: The limited growth span of cell strains isolated from the chick embryo. Exp. Gerontol. **2**, 123–135 (1967).

Hayflick, L., Moorhead, P. S.: The serial cultivation of human diploid cell strains. Exp. Cell Res. **25**, 585–621 (1961).

Hayflick, L.: The limited in vitro lifetime of human diploid cell strains. Exp. Cell Res. **37**, 614–636 (1965).

Hayflick, L.: Aging under glass. Exp. Gerontol. **5**, 291–303 (1970).

Hayflick, L.: Cell senescence and cell differentiation in vitro. Vol. 4, 1–15. In: H. Bredt and J. W. Rohen (Eds.), Aging and Development, F. K. Schattauer Verlag, Stuttgart, 1972.

Hayflick, L.: The biology of human aging. Am. J. Med. Sci. **265**, 433–445 (1973).

Hayflick, L.: The cell biology of human aging. N. Engl. J. Med. **295**, 1302–1308 (1976).

Hayflick, L.: The cellular basis for biological aging. In: C. Finch and L. Hayflick (Eds.), Handbook of the Biology of Aging. pp. 159−186. New York: Van Nostrand Reinhold, 1977.

Hayflick, L.: Cell Aging. In: C. Eisdorfer (Ed.), Annual Review of Gerontology and Geriatrics. pp. 26−67. New York: Springer, 1980.

Hellman, S., Botnick, L. E., Hannon, E. C., Vigneulle, R. M.: Proliferative capacity of murine hematopoietic stem cells. Proc. Nat. Acad. Sci. U.S.A. **75**, 490−494 (1978).

Krohn, P. L.: Review lectures on senescence. II: Heterochronic transplantation in the study of aging. Proc. R. Soc. Lond. [Biol.] **157**, 128−147 (1962).

LeGuilly, Y., Simon, M., Lenoir, P., Bourel, M.: Long-term culture of human adult liver cells: Morphological changes related to in vitro senescence and effect of donor's age on growth potential. Gerontologia **19**, 303−313 (1973).

Lesher, S., Fry, R. J. M., Kohn, H. I.: Age and the generation time of the mouse duodenal epithelial cell. Exp. Cell Res. **24**, 334−343 (1961a).

Lesher, S., Fry, R. J. M., Kohn, H. I.: Age and the generation cycle of intestinal epithelial cells in the mouse. Gerontologia (Basel) **5**, 176−181 (1961b).

Lesher, S., Sacher, G. A.: Effects of age on cell proliferation in mouse duodenal crypts. Exp. Gerontol. **3**, 211−217 (1968).

Martin, G. M., Sprague, C. A., Epstein, C. J.: Replicative lifespan of cultivated human cells. Effects of donor's age, tissue, and genotype. Lab. Invest. **23**, 86−92 (1970).

McHale, J. S., Moulton, M. L., McHale, J. T.: Limited culture lifespan of human diploid cells as a function of metabolic time instead of division potential. Exp. Gerontol. **6**, 89−93 (1971).

Nienhaus, A. J., DeJong, B., Tenkate, L. P.: Fibroblast culture in Werner's syndrome. Humangenetik **13**, 244−246 (1971).

Ogura, H., Fujawara, T., Namba, N.: Establishment of two chick embryo fibroblastic cell lines. Gann **75**, 410−414 (1984).

Reichel, W., Garcia-Bunuel, R., Dilallo, J.: Progeria and Werner's syndrome as models for the study of normal human aging. J. Am. Geriatr. Soc. **19**, 369−375 (1971).

Rohme, D.: Evidence for a relationship between longevity of mammalian species and lifespans of normal fibroblasts in vitro and erythrocytes in vivo. Proc. Nat. Acad. Sci. U.S.A. **78**, 5009−5013 (1981).

Schneider, E. L., Mitsui, Y.: The relationship between in vitro cellular aging and in vivo human age. Proc. Nat. Acad. Sci. U.S.A. **73**, 3584−3588 (1976).

Schneider, E. L., Mitsui, Y., Aw, K. S., Shorr, S.: Tissue-specific differences in cultured human diploid fibroblasts. Exp. Cell Res. **108**, 1−6 (1977).

Siminovitch, L., Till, J. E., McCulloch, E. A.: Decline in colony-forming ability of marrow cells subjected to serial transplantation into irradiated mice. J. Cell Comp. Physiol. **64**, 23−31 (1964).

Stanley, J. F., Pye, D., MacGregor, A.: Comparison of doubling numbers attained by cultured animal cells with the life span of species. Nature **255**, 158−159 (1975).

Stewart, H. L., Snell, K C., Dunham, L. J., Schylen, S. M.: Transplantable and transmissible tumors of animals. Washington, D.C., Armed Forces Institute of Pathology (1959).

Strebler, B. L., Mildvan, A. S.: General theory of mortality and aging. Science **132**, 14−21 (1960).

Tassin, J., Malaise, E., Courtois, Y.: Human lens cells have an in vitro proliferative capacity inversely proportional to the donor age. Exp. Cell Res. **129**, 345−350, 1979.

Thrasher, J. D., Greulich, R. C.: The duodenal progenitor population. I: Age related increase in the duration of the cryptal progenitor cycle. J. Exp. Zool. **159**, 39−46 (1965).

Till, J. E., McCulloch, E. A., Siminovitch, L.: Isolation of variant cell lines during serial transplantation of hematopoietic cells derived from fetal liver. J. Nat. Cancer Inst. **33**, 707−720 (1964).

Vracko, R., McFarland, B. M.: Lifespan of diabetic and non-diabetic fibroblasts in vitro. Exp. Cell Res. **129**, 345−350 (1980).

Walford, R. L., Jawaid, S. Q., Naeim, F.: Evidence for in vitro senescence of T-lymphocytes cultured from normal human peripheral blood. Age **4**, 67−70 (1981).

Walford, R. L.: Studies on immunogerontology. J. Am. Geriat. Soc. **30**, 617−625 (1982).

Williamson, A. R., Askonas, B. A.: Senescence of an antibody-forming cell clone. Nature **238**, 337−339 (1972).

Williamson, A. R.: Extent and control of antibody diversity. Biochem. J. **130**, 325−333 (1972).

Witkowski, J. A.: The myth of cell immortality. Trends in Biochem. Sci. **10**, 258−260 (1985).

Young, L. J. T., Medina, D., deOme, K. B., Daniel, C. W.: The influence of host and tissue age on the lifespan and growth rate of serially transplanted mouse mammary gland. Exp. Gerontol. **6**, 49−56 (1971).

Drug Compliance in the Elderly

M. J. Denham

Northwick Park Hospital and Clinical Research Center, Watford Road, Harrow, Middlesex
HA1 3UJ, U.K.

Introduction

Since the Second World War there has been a pharmaceutical revolution both in the
variety and range of medications which are now available. This has brought immense
benefit to patients of all ages including the elderly. These benefits have been 'bought'
at the expense of an increase in adverse drug reactions in older people (referred to later
in the symposium) and also in financial expenditure.

The cost of the pharmaceutical service in the United Kingdom is currently about £ 1600
million a year (Office of Health Economics — OHE 1984). This considerable sum is
spent on a variety of drugs. The most popular prescribed medicines for patients of all
ages in 1970 were hypnotics, expectorants, minor analgesics, sedatives and penicillin,
but in 1982, diuretics, topical skin preparations, sedatives and tranquillisers were the
most commonly prescribed (Table I). Unfortunately there are no nationally available
statistics which rank drugs according to prescribing practice to the older person. However
Christopher and colleagues (1978) analysed the prescribing practice of hospital doctors
in a large district general hospital in respect of the elderly in geriatric, psychiatric, medical, surgical and orthopaedic wards. The most commonly prescribed medicines were
hypnotics, sedatives, laxatives, diuretics and potassium supplements (Table II). Community prescribing for the elderly appears somewhat different. Williamson and Chopin
(1980) found that elderly people admitted to geriatric wards from home had been most
frequently prescribed diuretics, analgesics, as well as a vast range of drugs acting on the
central nervous system. It is interesting to note that in my own hospital, prescribing
costs for patients in geriatric wards and in the geriatric out-patient department amounts
to 5% of the district pharmaceutical budget, with most money being spent on anti-

Table I: The most frequently prescribed drug preparations in the United Kingdom in
1970 and 1982 (OHE 1984)

1970	1982
Hypnotics	Diuretics
Expectorants and Cough Suppresants	Topical Skin Preparations
Analgesics Minor	Sedatives and Tranquillisers
Sedatives and Tranquillisers	Analgesics Minor
Penicillins	Penicillins
Tetracyclines	Heart Preparations
Antacids	Anti-Inflammatory Preparations

Table II: Principal drug groups prescribed to the elderly (n = number of patients studied)

Christopher et al. 1978 (n = 873)	Williamson and Chopin 1980 (n = 1998)
Neuroleptics	Diuretics
Chloral Derivatives	Analgesics
Diuretics	Antidepressants, Tranquillisers and Psychomimetics
Laxatives	Hypnotics and Sedatives
Mineral Supplements	Digitalis
Analgesics	Salts (K)

microbial medicines, drugs which act on the central nervous system and those which heal gastro-intestinal ulcers. As might be expected, more is spent on patients in the admitting wards relative to those in rehabilitation and long-stay wards.

Disproportionate Prescribing in the Elderly

The elderly are given more medication than younger people since doctors naturally wish to do all they can to alleviate the increasing disability and disease which tend to occur in older people. In 1980 the elderly were given twice as many prescriptions as the national average (OHE 1984). Dunnell and Cartwright (1972) showed a steady increase in the number of prescribed medicines relative to age, although curiously perhaps, the taking of over the counter preparations remained fairly constant throughout life. Williamson and Chopin (1980) found that 80% of elderly patients admitted to hospital had been receiving medicines while in the community, a figure similar to that found by Moir and Dingwall-Fordyce (1980) in their community study. This high rate of prescribing is not parallelled by a similar high consultation rate with the local general practitioner. This may be due to the elderly having a more stoical attitude to infirmity combined with a tendency to attribute potentially treatable ailments to the ageing process. In addition there is a tendency for multiple repeat prescriptions to replace consultations and the elderly often find it difficult to visit the general practitioners' surgeries.

Compliance in the Elderly

Compliance studies of elderly people have shown that as many as three-quarters of them make errors in their medication and a quarter of these are potentially serious (Schwartz et al. 1962, MacDonald et al. 1977). However older people seem to be less likely to make errors with drugs which they buy over the counter (Kiernan and Isaacs 1981).

Measurement of Compliance

To understand the problem of compliance it is helpful to review the various methods by which it can be measured. There are two basic techniques — the direct and indirect. The direct method involves the measurement in blood or urine of the drug, its metabolite or a marker. Because of problems of chemical analysis, only a few drugs, such as digoxin, anti-biotics, anti-hypertensive and anti-epileptic drugs, are measured in this way. The value of the technique is also limited by the rate at which drugs are eliminated. The measurement of the blood concentration of a drug which has a long half life can indicate compliance over preceding weeks but the measurement of the blood concentration of a drug with a short half life may indicate only whether the previous dose has been taken or not. The same problem applies to measurement of drugs in urine.

Four indirect methods of assessing compliance are frequently used in preference to the direct technique because of the problems mentioned above.

(i) Firstly there is the tablet count. If the number of tablets prescribed to the patient, as well as the number in the patient's possession, are known, then it is possible to calculate the number of tablets which it is assumed the patient has taken. However people do sometimes share their tablets with others, and some have been known to dispose of the relevant number of tablets in order to make the tablet count come out correctly (Porter 1969). Another problem with this method is that it does not detect altered patterns of compliance, e.g. a person may take more tablets during one week than the next.

(ii) The second method involves patient interviews. This allows the doctor to identify the problem and hopefully correct them but it clearly depends on truthful answers, e.g. some psychiatric patients have said they have been taking their drugs correctly although urine tests have shown a complete absence of the appropriate medication (Willcox et al. 1965).

(iii) The third method involves the assessment of demands for new supplies of medication. This is not as helpful as might be expected, and it may act as a cloak for hoarding. A 71 year old gentleman was admitted to hospital some years ago with an attempted overdose. He was found to have in his possession 10,685 tablets and capsules which had been prescribed to him over the preceding 17 months (Smith and Stead 1974).

(iv) The fourth method involves assessment of clinical outcome but this may not always be easy to establish.

Consequently it is not entirely surprising that there is no universally agreed or accepted method of assessing compliance.

Causes of Poor Compliance

In spite of the problems of assessing compliance it does seem that three groups of patients, the elderly, the confused and those on long-term medication, are those most likely to make mistakes in their drug taking, although other sensible people are also found to default on occasion.

1. *The Patient*: Several studies have shown decreasing compliance associated with increasing age and impaired mental state (Schwartz et al. 1962, Boyd et al. 1974, MacDonald et al. 1977). However there is no correlation between compliance and sex, and various social factors such as occupation, income, religion and education. Compliance does tend to deteriorate in those who live alone and those who are said to 'not to cope very well at home' (Schwartz et al. 1962, Parkin et al. 1976).

2. *The Illness*: The patient's perception of his illness can result in him/her making a positive decision to stop taking the medicine. The factors here include a total lack of symptoms, early disappearance of symptoms, lack of response to treatment and a lack of faith in the doctor (Sackett et al. 1975, Hemminski and Heikkila 1975).

3. *The Physician*: The Physician is responsible for the quality of the explanation to the patient about how and when to take the medicines, and also responsible for the quality

Table III: Extent of dose variation related to dose frequency in 198 preparations (Kiernan and Isaacs 1981)

Frequency of dose	Number of Drugs Variation from correct dose (%)	Total
One tablet morning only	1 (6)	18
One tablet evening only	4 (29)	14
One tablet twice a day	4 (31)	13
One tablet three times a day	15 (75)	20
Other regimes	72 (54)	133

of the prescription given to the Pharmacist. There clearly are occasions when physicians fail to give adequate instructions. Thus patients have failed to comply and on occasion have reverted to the dosages prescribed to them before they came into hospital (Parkin et al. 1976, Kiernan and Isaacs 1981). However sometimes basic knowledge is assumed to be present but which is found to be absent on subsequent investigation. A study of the use of suppositories showed that half the patients concerned failed to take the wrapper off before inserting them into the rectum (Wootton 1975).

Doctors can complicate the problem of compliance by completing inadequately the prescription form which is to be taken to the pharmacist. If the form only indicates the strength and number of tablets, the pharmacist is likely to write on the instruction label 'to be taken as directed'.

4. The Treatment: The number and timing of the drugs to be taken is important. The more drugs given per day and the more complex the regime the worse the compliance. Drugs which need to be taken more than twice a day are difficult to fit into a day time schedule and mistakes are increasingly likely (Table III). Also, patients seem less likely to take greasy skin preparations, drugs which cause unpleasant side effects, and suppositories, but seem to have a higher level of compliance for drugs which act on the cardiovascular system (Drury et al. 1976, Parkin et al. 1976).

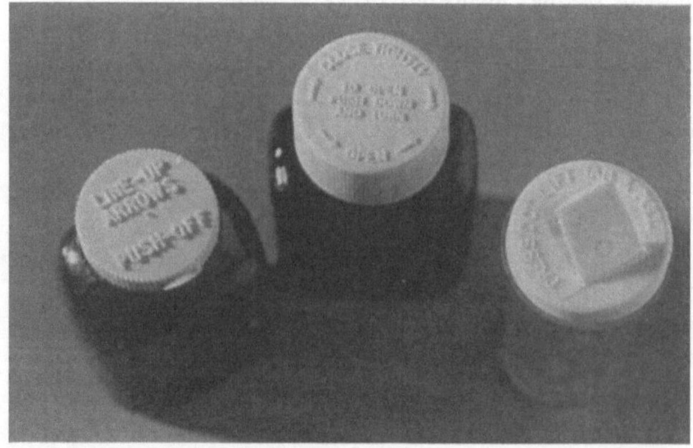

Fig. 1
Examples of child resistant containers

5. *The Pharmacist*: The labelling on the drug container is most important. Over the counter preparations are more likely to have printed labels which are legible, but patients may well have difficulty in reading badly written labels on prescribed medicines. As many as a half of a group of elderly people living in the community were unable to read the labels on their drug containers (Jenkins 1979, Kiernan and Isaacs 1981).

Since the elderly may have impaired eye-sight and manual dexterity, care has to be taken to ensure that the patient can open the drug bottle or container. The situation has been compounded within recent years following the introduction of child resistant containers which aim to reduce the risk of accidental overdose in children. Typical examples are the click-lock, pop-lock and snap-safe bottles (Fig. 1). The inability of old people to open these containers, particularly the click-lock, is now well recognised. It has been suggested that the elderly might find blister, bubble or strip pack containers easier to manage but this has not proved to be the case (Davidson 1973).

The Dangers of Non-Compliance

Poor compliance can have serious effects on the patient and his illness, sometimes with repercussions on the community. Those most at risk are those on drugs with a narrow therapeutic range and those in whom loss of control of the disease is serious, for example diabetic, epileptic or tuberculous patients.

Poor compliance or mis-prescribing can result in hoarding (Fig. 2) which can be extensive. Consequently, from time to time in the United Kingdom campaigns are carried out to arrange the Disposal of Unwanted Medicines and Poisons (DUMP). A recent campaign in Glasgow produced two and a quarter tons of unwanted medicines. A similar campaign in Birmingham (Harris et al. 1979) produced a third of a million tablets/capsules but this was calculated to represent only 3% of the potential total. The majority of drugs returned were diuretics, respiratory medicines, analgesics and antibiotics. There was strong evidence that only half of the courses of antibiotics had been taken. Over 70% of the drugs were over one year old and some showed definite signs of deterioration.

There are three potential serious consequences of drug hoarding. Firstly, the patient may confuse the bottles of newly prescribed drugs with the hoarded ones, leading to

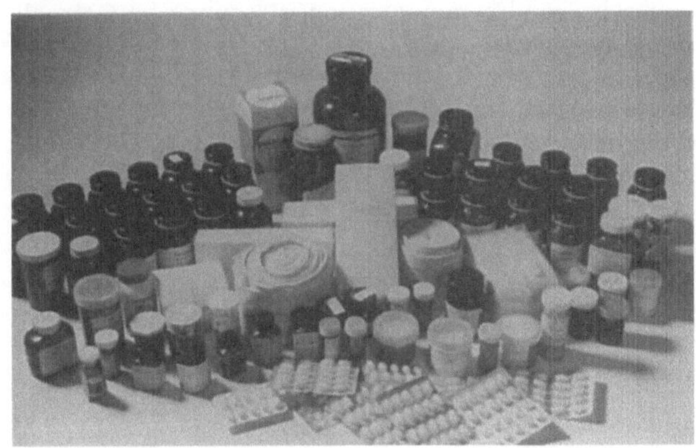

Fig. 2

Example of hoarding of medicines by an elderly person

inappropriate dose/drug schedule. In addition drugs may be shared with others. Secondly, some drugs deteriorate with age, e.g. glyceryl trinitrate which lasts only 6—8 weeks before becoming ineffective. Thirdly, patients may use hoarded drugs inappropriately. A man kept a bottle of steroid eye drops which had been prescribed for his iritis. He used the drug again when he subsequently developed further pain in his eye. Unfortunately his new symptom was due to a dendritic ulcer with the result that he perforated his cornea and required an emergency corneal graft.

Measures to Improve Compliance

Several methods can be used to improve compliance by making it mentally simpler for the patient to understand the drug regime and physically easier to take the tablets. The results of such measures varies.

1. Medication Regime: The medication regime must be made as simple as possible, giving as few drugs as possible during the day, with doses related to meal times or other regular activities. Although the combination of drugs into one tablet has many known disadvantages, it may be helpful in this situation.

2. Patient Instruction and Counselling: Compliance is likely to improve when patients are given simple, clear instructions repeated over a period of time. If this is combined with an explanation of the need for the therapy and enquiries about problems with taking tablets, then compliance may be maintained at a reasonable level for some time.

3. Written Information: Written instructions coupled with drug record cards can usefully support verbal instructions.

4. Containers: It seems likely that clear-coloured glass, screw or snap-topped containers are best for older people since they are easier to open and enable the medicine to be identified by colour (Davidson 1973). For the arthritic person, containers with winged tops are helpful.

5. Labelling: Clear, explicit labels are required which should be printed in large letters or typewritten. Vague instructions such as 'to be taken as directed' should be avoided where at all possible.

6. Memory Aids: A number of different aids are available to help compliance. The Dosette box (Fig. 3) is widely used but does require someone to fill it once a week and unfortunately it is not child-proof. Calender packs can be helpful.

7. Supervision and Long-Term Medication: Many elderly people are responsible for taking their own medicines. Consequently, good communication is required between all caring staff regarding a patient's drugs and relevant doses. Adequate follow-up is necessary in the patient's home, doctor's surgery, or the hospital out-patient department. The patient should always be asked to bring his/her tablets to the surgery or out-patient department in order to check that the drug regime is understood. In order to reduce the problem of unchecked repeat prescriptions, it is helpful if general practitioners 'flag' the patient's prescription card so that the medication regime is reviewed after a certain number of repeats.

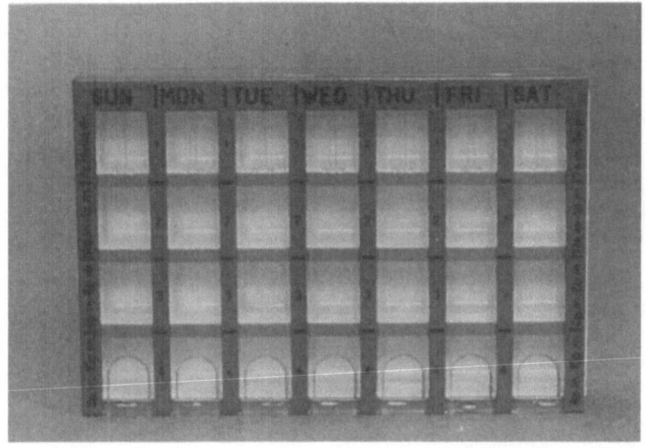

Fig. 3
Memory Aid — A Dosette box

Conclusion

Drug compliance is likely to improve if the drug regime is kept as simple as possible using as few drugs as possible each day. Clear, reinforced explanations supported by written instructions using precise well-labelled clear-coloured containers will also be helpful. The judicious use of special memory aids may be useful. Adequate follow-up should always be arranged and care taken to avoid unnecessary repeat prescriptions.

References

Boyd, J. R., Covington, T. R., Stanaszeh, W. F., Coussons, T. T.: Drug defaulting Part II. Analysis of non compliance patterns. American Journal of Hospital Pharmacy **31**, 485, 1974

Christopher, L. J., Ballinger, B. R., Shepherd, A. M. M., Ramsay, A., Crooks, G.: Drug prescribing patterns in the elderly: a cross sectional study of in-patients. Age and Ageing **7**, 74, 1978

Davidson, J. R.: Presentation and Packaging of drugs for the elderly. Journal of Hospital Pharmacy **31**, 180, 1973

Drury, V. S. M., Wade, O. L., Woolf, E.: Following advice in general practice. Journal of Royal College of General Practitioners **26**, 712, 1976

Dunnell, K., Cartwright, A.: Medicine taken, prescribed and hoarded. London: Routledge, Kegan and Paul, 1972

Harris, D. W., Karandikar, D. S., Spencer, M. G., Leach, R. H., Bower, A. C., Mander, G. A.: Returned medicine campaign in Birmingham in 1977, Lancet **1**, 599, 1979

Hemminki, E., Heikkila, J.: Elderly people's compliance with prescriptions and quality of medication. Scandinavian Journal of Social Medicine **3**, 87, 1975

Jenkins, G. H. C.: Drug compliance and the elderly patients. British Medical Journal **1**, 124, 1979

Kiernan, P. J., Isaacs, J. B.: Use of drugs by the elderly. Journal of Royal Society of Medicine **74**, 196, 1981

MacDonald, E. T., MacDonald, J. B., Phoenix, M.: Improving drug compliance after hospital discharge. British Medical Journal **2**, 618, 1977

Moir, D. C., Dingwall-Fordyce, I.: Drug taking in the elderly at home. Journal of Clinical and Experimental Gerontology **2**, 329, 1980

Office of Health Economics: Compendium of Health Statistics (Section of Pharmaceutical Services) 5th edition London, 1984

Parkin, D. M., Henney, C. R., Quirk, J., Crooks, J.: Deviation from prescribed drug treatment after discharge from hospital. British Medical Journal **2**, 686, 1976

Porter, A. M.: Drug defaulting in general practice. British Medical Journal **1**, 218, 1969

Sackett, D. C., Haynes, R. B., Gibson, E. S., Hackett, B. C., Tayler, D. W., Robert, R. S., Johnson, A. L.: Randomised clinical trials of strategies for improving compliance in hypertension. Lancet **1**, 1205, 1975

Schwartz, D., Wang, M., Zeitz, L., Goss, M. E. W.: Medication errors made by elderly chronically ill patients. American Journal of Public Health **52**, 2018, 1962

Smith, S. E., Stead, K. C.: Non-compliance or mis-prescribing. Lancet **1**, 937, 1974

Willcox, D. R. G., Gilles, R., Hare, E. H.: Do psychiatric patients take their drugs. British Medical Journal **2**, 790, 1965

Williamson, J., Chopin, J. M.: Adverse drug reactions to prescribed drugs in the elderly: a multicentre investigation. Age and Ageing **9**, 73, 1980

Wootton, J.: Prescription for error. Nursing Times **71**, 884, 1975

Adverse Drug Reactions in Elderly Patients

C. M. Castleden
Leicester General Hospital Leicester, UK

Summary

This paper argues that the high number of adverse drugs reactions (ADR) in elderly patients results mostly from their increased use of drugs. This is due to their multiple pathology and symptomatology. Altered drug kinetics and dynamics with ageing are relatively minor causes of ADR's. Thus a major reduction in ADR's in this age group would only follow a reduction in prescription rate and the length of treatment. Nevertheless, doctors should still critically review dosage and rely on clinical observation of effect as the maxim for using larger doses.

The Problem

There is no argument that the number of ADR's increases with the number of drugs taken [1], nor is there any doubt that ADR's cause a singnificant morbidity and mortality in the elderly. Before the late 1960's, ADR publications in this age group consisted largely of case reports. Since that time, however, several centres have individually shown a positive correlation between the number of ADR's and ageing [2, 3, 4]. The Bosten Colaborative Drug Surveillance Programme has specifically identified individual drugs such as Diazepam, Flurazepam, Nitrazepam and Heparin in this respect [5]. Smith and Haber [6] had reported earlier on the association between Digoxin toxicity and ageing although such toxicity was more clearly related to renal function which is known to decrease in the elderly.

Williamson [7] found that 12.4% of elderly patients admitted to hospital suffered an ADR although the nature of the reaction was not defined. He also took no account of self purchased medication which is a large component of an elderly patient's drug therapy. Nevertheless, an ADR was the sole cause of admission in 2.5%, and a contributory cause in 7.7%. Most importantly he found that a substantial number did not recover fully after their ADR although ADR's seem to cause deaths only in severely ill patients [8].

A substantial drawback of all these reports is that they are hospital based and largely conducted from medical wards. This does not detract from their conclusions, but clearly age is not the sole factor, frequently being swamped by the severity and duration of disease. Medical patients are on the whole older than those in other specialities, and elderly patients go to Hospital more frequently because of ADR's.

The Cause

Explanations for the increased numbers of ADR's in elderly patients include increased severity of illness, altered kinetics and dynamics with ageing per se, and multiple diseases and therefore symptoms demanding an increased number of drugs. Any review of prescription figures allows one to sympathize with the old lady who said she no longer had a doctor looking after her but only a man who sent her pills. Williamson [7] reported that the top five groups of drugs of patients admitted to Geriatric Departments were diuretics (37.4%), Analgesics (27.4%), antidepressants, tranquillizers and psychominetics (23.7%), hypnotics, sedatives and anticonvulsants (22.2%), and Digoxin preparations (20.1%) and that the greatest number of reactions occurred with those drugs most frequently used. Thus diuretics were responsible for the highest number of ADR's with psychotropics a close second. The sole exception seems to be analgesics which caused comparatively few ADR's. However, it is not just the total number of drugs but also that the type and class of drug changes with ageing. Castleden and George [9] found that the elderly living in the Community were two and a half times more likely to take drugs known to interact adversely with other therapy and Williamson found that the risk of an ADR was highest with hypotensive, Parkinsonian, antidepressant and Digoxin therapy, (only 4% of the elderly in Castleden and Georges' survey were on such drugs). The present hypothesis is that if the younger patients were given the same types of drug as the older in the same numbers, they would have the same ADR rate. Recent evidence from the CSM on the rate of ADR's compared to the number of prescriptions of non-steroidal anti-inflammatory drugs corroborates this hypothesis.

If the total number of drugs is important then clearly so is the duration of treatment. Not only because it governs the patient's drug exposure and possible interaction with other medication but also because the development of some ADR's is clearly related to the duration of treatment, such as tardive dyskinesia following phenothiazine therapy.

An increase in ADR's in elderly patients is seen with increasing dosage with some drugs, eg, Nitrazepam [10] and Flurazepam [11], but these elderly were hospitalised and may well have been iller than the young [12]. It is unlikely that many ADR's result from kinetic or dynamic changes with ageing per se since they are so easily swamped by disease and other factors such as smoking and alcohol ingestion [13]. Even when researchers attempt to hold other factors steady so that they may examine the effects of ageing on drug kinetics or dynamics many other variables are included inevitably. Why the elderly especially females suffer more from marrow depression following co-trimoxazole [14] and phenylbutazone [15] is unknown but may represent folate deficiency rather than a true ageing phenomenon.

A failure to comply with medical instructions is frequently cited as a cause of ADR's in elderly patients. However, the most common sin is that of omission [16], and thus confusion is unlikely to be a major cause of ADR's in this age group.

The Solution

Clearly ADR's are related to the number of drugs taken and thus it is more important for doctors to worry about the actual numbers, length of treatment and advice on self medication than on the correct dosage for elderly patients. This is not to dismiss dosage as unimportant but rather not to elevate it to such an extent that doctors fail to recognise the prime factor in causing an increased number of ADR's in elderly patients. Furthermore, dosage for elderly patients largely follows that for younger patients with the same diseases, (for example, Digoxin in renal failure) rather than any special guidelines, and doctors cannot do better than follow the maxim that increases in dose should only follow clinical observation of the effect of a smaller one.

There are special cases in which special care is necessary such as patients with previous drug reaction and those severely ill. There are also the marrow reactions that follow certain drugs. The mechanism for which is unexplained as yet, but alternative drugs are available in every class so far incriminated.

In conclusion, it is rare for an elderly patient to be taking no drugs but this author does not advocate therapeutic nihilism. The undoubted benefits of drug therapy are clear to both patients and doctors; the aim is to decrease any harm such drugs do to a minority of patients by taking care at the time of prescription. A doctor should ask himself: is this drug necessary, what is the shortest time I can give it, what other drugs are the patients taking, have I counselled her on self medication, what dose shall I use and when will I see her again to review the effect of this drug?

References

[1] Cliff, L.E., Thornton, G.F., Seidl, L.G.: Studies on the epidemiology of adverse drug reactions. JAMA. **188**, 976−983 (1964).

[2] Hurwitz, N., Wade, O. L.: Intensive hospital monitoring of adverse reactions to drugs. Br. Med. J. **1**, 531−536 (1969).

[3] Ogilvie, R. I., Ruedy, J.: Adverse drug reactions during hospitalization. Can. Med. Ass. J. **97**, 1450−1457 (1967).

[4] Seidly, L. G., Thornton, G. F., Smith, J. W., Cliff, L. E.: Studies on the epidemology of adverse drug reactions. III reactions in patients on a general medical service. John Hopkins Hospital Bul. **119**, 299−315 (1966).

[5] Koch-Weser, J.,Greenblatt, D. S., Sellers, E. M., Shader, R. I.: Drug disposition in old age. New Eng. J. Med. **306**, 1081−1082 (1982).

[6] Smith, T. W., Haber, E.: Digoxin intoxication: the relationship of clinical presentation to serum digoxin concentration. J. Clin. Invest. **49**, 2377−2386 (1970).

[7] Williamson, J., Chopin, J. M.: Adverse reactions to prescribed drugs in the elderly: a multi-centre investigations. Age and Ageing **9**, 73−80 (1980).

[8] Jue, S. G., Vestal, R. E.: Adverse drug reactions in the elderly in clinical pharmacology and drug treatment in the elderly. Ed. K. O'Malley, Churchill Livingstone, P52−70 (1984).

[9] Castleden, C. M., George, C. F.: Prescription for the elderly in clinical pharmacology and drug treatment in the elderly. Ed. K. O'Malley, Churchill Livingstone, P71−98 (1984).

[10] Greenblatt, D. J., Allen, M. D.: Toxicity of nitrazepam in the elderly. Br. J. Clin. Pharmacol. **5**, 407−13 (1978).

[11] Greenblatt, D. J., Allen, M. D., Shader, R. I.: Toxicity of high-dose flurazepam in the elderly. Clinic. Pharmacol. Ther. **21**, 355−61 (1977).

[12] Castleden, C. M.: The use of hypnotics in elderly patients with impaired liver function. In: Liver and Ageing, Ed. K. Kitani, Elsevier Biomedical Press. P331−346 (1982).

[13] Wood, A. J. J., Vestal, R. E., Wilkinson, G. R., Branch, R. A., Shand, D. G.: Effect of ageing and cigarette smoking on antipyrine and indocyanine green elimination. Clin. Pharmacol. and Ther. **26**, 16−20 (1979).

[14] Committee on safety of medicines: Current Problems, No 15 (1985).

[15] Inman, W. H. W.: Study of fatal bone marrow depression with special reference to phenylbutazone. Br. Med. J. **1**, 1500−1505 (1977).

[16] Law, R., Chalmers, C.: Medicines in elderly people: a general practice survey. Brit. Med. J. **1**, 565−568 (1976).

II Effect of Age on Pharmacodynamics and Drug Disposition

Drug Distribution and Pharmacologic Effect: Relation to Drug Therapy in the Elderly

D. J. Greenblatt
Division of Clinical Pharmacology, Box 1007
Tufts-New England Medical Center, 171 Harrison Avenue, Boston, MA 02111, USA

Summary

Pharmacokinetic studies of drug disposition in old age so far have emphasized age-related changes in elimination and clearance. However, alterations in body habitus associated with the aging process can lead to changes in patterns of drug distribution, which are independent of changes in clearance. Since drug distribution, rather than drug clearance, may be the most important determinant of the time-course and intensity of pharmacologic action after single doses, altered drug distribution in the elderly may contribute to age-related changes in clinical drug activity particularly after single doses.

Because the proportion of elderly individuals among the population of Western nations is continuously increasing, health care delivery increasingly involves the pharmacotherapy of medical disease in the geriatric population. Many experimental and pharmacologic studies, as well as extensive clinical experience, indicates that aging individuals may have altered sensitivity to a number of pharmacologic agents (Greenblatt et al, 1982a; Schmucker, 1985; Vestal, 1982; Sjöqvist and Alvan, 1983). Usually the elderly manifest increased drug sensitivity, evident clinically as a greater likelihood of excessive drug effects or adverse reactions at what are usually considered "therapeutic" doses. In a few cases, reduced drug sensitivity in the elderly has been described (Vestal et al, 1979). Basic and clinical research has focused on the mechanisms underlying altered drug sensitivity in the elderly. This change appears to be explained by age-related alterations in intrinsic receptor sensitivity, as well as by altered drug clearance leading to different steady-state drug concentrations at any given dosing rate.

Most studies of drug disposition in the elderly have focused on alterations in drug biotransformation, elimination, and clearance. The steady-state serum or plasma concentration of a drug during multiple dosage (Css) is directly related to the dosing rate (the rate at which the drug is administered), as well as the drug's total clearance, according to the following equation:

$$\text{Css} = \frac{\text{Dosing rate}}{\text{Clearance}} \ . \tag{1}$$

The validity of this relationship underlies the importance of understanding alterations in drug clearance among elderly individuals. Although health care professionals have control over dosing rate, clearance is a biologically determined variable, giving in numerical terms the capacity of a given individual to remove a given drug (Greenblatt and Koch-Weser, 1975; Greenblatt and Shader, 1985). Since clearance is in the denominator of Eq. (1), reductions in clearance associated with the aging process will lead to elevations in Css, and an increased potential for drug toxicity, unless dosing rate is appropriately adjusted. Thus understanding of alterations in drug clearance in the elderly assumes primary importance during the multiple dosing situation during which steady-state has been reached.

However, many drugs are not taken on a chronic basis, but are rather taken as isolated single doses, or as single doses at widely spaced intervals. This is often true for medications such as analgesics or hypnotics. Under these circumstances, the major determinant of the time-course and intensity of clinical response is not necessarily clearance, but rather the rate and extent of drug distribution. Considerable research has focused on alterations in drug clearance associated with the aging process, but less attention has been paid to changes in drug distribution in the elderly, which may be equally or more striking than alterations in clearance.

This paper reviews the concept of drug distribution, its pharmacokinetic measurement, and its possible clinical consequences for drug therapy in the elderly.

The Pharmacokinetics of Drug Distribution

The pharmacokinetic concept of volume of distribution derives from the definition of concentration (Greenblatt and Shader, 1985). If a given amount or quantity of a drug is homogeneously dissolved in a solution having a specified volume, then its concentration in that solution can be defined as:

$$\text{Concentration} = \frac{\text{Amount}}{\text{Volume}} . \tag{2}$$

In the living organism, two of these three variables can be either measured or inferred with reasonable accuracy. If a given dose (D) of a drug is administered and if the time elapsing after dosage is not long enough for a significant amount of the drug to be biotransformed or excreted, then the amount of the drug present in the body is approximately equal to the administered dose. The drug concentration in a body fluid — usually blood, serum, or plasma — can then be measured with reasonable accuracy using appropriate techniques of analytical chemistry. In Eq. (2), amount and concentration are the "known" quantities, whereas volume is unknown. The pharmacokinetic definition of volume of distribution (Vd) comes from the rearrangement of Eq. (2) to calculate the unknown quantity:

$$Vd = \frac{\text{amount}}{\text{concentration}} . \tag{3}$$

Thus pharmacokinetic volume of distribution has units of volume (liters or mililiters) and is derived from known values of amount and concentration. The pharmacokinetic Vd is an imaginary volume, and is not actually the volume of any particular tissue or combination of tissues; that is, it is not really the volume of "anything". Nonetheless, Vd conceptually useful, since it gives an idea of the extent of drug distribution within the living organism. Consider, for example, a drug such as diazepam. A typical clinical situation is that the amount of diazepam in the body is 10 mg, while the measured concentration in serum or plasma is 0.1 μg/ml. From Eq. (3), the calculated pharmacokinetic Vd for diazepam is 100 liters. Since this is larger than the actual volume of a typically sized human volunteer or patient (i.e., 70 kg) in which such studies are performed (Greenblatt et al, 1980), the fictitious nature of Vd is thereby illustrated. Nonetheless, Vd is a useful quantitative estimate of the extent of diazepam distribution in vivo. The Vd value of 100 liters implies that, if the concentration of diazepam throughout the body were homogeneous, the total volume of the body compartment would have to be 100 liters in order to account for the low concentration present in plasma. In biologic terms, this Vd value illustrates that the actual concentration of diazepam in some body compartments must considerably exceed those present in plasma. Actual tissue uptake studies of diazepam, both in animals and humans, verify that its concentrations in many tissues exceed those in plasma (Friedman et al, 1985a, 1985b, 1985c; Greenblatt and Arendt, 1985). This is commonly observed for lipophilic (lipid-soluble) drugs: their pharmacokinetic Vd values exceed the actual size of the body. For relatively water soluble drugs and/or those that are extensively bound to plasma protein (such as ibuprofen, salicylate, and other non-steroidal antiinflammatory agents), Vd values as small as 10 to 15% of body weight have been reported in pharmacokinetic studies (Greenblatt et al, 1984, 1985; Verbeeck et al, 1983). Values such as these indicate minimal drug uptake into extravascular tissues, and that most of the drug present in the body is confined to the intravascular compartment.

The Quantitation of Volume of Distribution

When drug behavior within the body is consistent with a single homogeneous pharmacokinetic compartment, then a single Vd value correctly serves as a proportionality constant between the amount of drug in the body and the concentration in a reference compartment (Eq. (3)). For the one compartment model, therefore, Vd is unique, and there is no controversy about the method of its calculation. Unfortunately a one compartment model adequately describes the in vivo behavior of relatively few drugs. For most drugs, disposition in the living organism is consistent with a pharmacokinetic model having two or more distinct compartments. In such cases, the drug will disappear from plasma in biphasic fashion following a rapid intravenous bolus, mathematically consistent with a linear sum of two or more exponential terms. Furthermore, no single value of Vd correctly serves as a proportionality constant between plasma concentration and amount of drug in the body at all times after drug administration. The two most common approaches to calculating Vd for such a pharmacokinetic model are the steady-state method and the area (or beta) method. Although Vd by the steady-state method is often assumed to be the most appropriate and "physiologically pure" volume parameter (Klotz, 1976), this assumption is incorrect and is unsupported by objective experimental evidence (Greenblatt et al, 1983a). The limitations and drawbacks of Vd by the steady-state method are as follows:

1. It serves as a correct proportionality constant between amount of drug in the body and concentration in plasma (Eq. (3)) at only a single instant in time following a rapid intravenous injection of a drug.

2. Its mathematical estimation is very dependent on the precise configuration of the initial phase of the plasma concentration curve, which is exceedingly difficult to determine in actual experimental studies, owing to inherent limitations in the precision of sample timing and withdrawal (Chiou, 1980; Chiou et al, 1981; Niazi, 1976). Small variations in the configuration of this part of the curve, due to methodologic problems or to other unknown reasons, can lead to large variations in estimates of Vd by the steady-state method.

Vd calculated by the area or beta method, on other hand, has distinct advantages as a volume estimate. These are:

1. It correctly serves as a proportionality constant between amount of drug in the body and plasma concentration at all points in time after distribution equilibrium has been attained.
2. It is essentially independent of unpredictable variations in the initial phase of the serum concentration curve following rapid intravenous injection. Therefore it is a "stable" pharmacokinetic parameter, which varies very little from time to time on repeated administration of a given drug to a given individual.

It is also commonly assumed that Vd by the steady-state method is a volume estimate that is "independent" of elimination processes. Vd by the area method, on the other hand, is stated to be dependent on drug elimination. Again, this assumption is incorrect, and is unsupported by scientific evidence (Greenblatt et al, 1983a). A number of studies in fact demonstrate that elimination half-life in the post-distributional phase of the plasma concentration curve is a dependent variable, being directly related to Vd and inversely related to clearance as follows:

$$\text{half-life} = \frac{0.693 \times \text{Vd}}{\text{clearance}} . \tag{4}$$

This relationship correctly depicts the dependent biologic variable on the left of the equation, and the two independent variables on the right of the equation. Elimination half-life is biologically dependent on Vd, and not the reverse; this dependence can be demonstrated whether Vd is measured by the steady-state method or the area method. The relationship has been shown in pharmacokinetic studies of physiologic states that lead to altered drug distribution without an alteration in clearance. An example is morbid obesity, which can cause large increases in Vd of lipophilic drugs without changing their clearance (Abernethy and Greenblatt, 1982). In such cases, elimination half-life increases in direct proportion to Vd, regardless of how Vd is measured. Thus elimination half-life is dependent on Vd, and not the reverse.

More extensive discussion can be found in a previous review (Greenblatt et al, 1983a).

Determinants of Drug Distribution

For most drugs, distribution within the living organism is a "passive" process, governed by first order kinetics and well-described principles of diffusion. Not surprisingly, in vivo Vd depends in large part on a given drug's propensity to be taken up into the various tissues of the body. This, in turn, depends on the drug's solubility in individual tissues. Since lipid is a component of many tissues (most obviously adipose tissue), it is further logical that drug uptake into tissues is related to its physicochemical properties of lipid solubility. This physicochemical characteristic can be measured in vitro, either by the drug's partition coefficient between an organic solvent (usually octanol) and an aqueous phase, or by its retention on a reverse-phase high pressure liquid chromatography (HPLC) system (Greenblatt et al, 1983b; Arendt et al, 1983). Highly lipid soluble drugs, for example, yield very high octanol:water partition ratios, and have long retention times on an appropriate HPLC system. Relatively water soluble drugs, on the other hand, have low octanol:water partition ratios, and are retained for only a short time on the HPLC system. A number of studies have indicated that in vivo Vd of drugs can be largely explained by or correlated with in vitro properties of lipid solubility (Ritschel and Hammer, 1980; Greenblatt et al, 1983b; Arendt et al, 1983; Ochs et al, 1985). This has been demonstrated not only for the pharmacokinetic Vd, but also for the actual measured extent of tissue uptake (Greenblatt and Arendt, 1985; Friedman et al, 1985b, 1985c).

In physiologic conditions in which adipose tissue is increased relative to lean body mass, the Vd of drugs can change dramatically. In individuals with morbid obesity, highly lipophilic drugs such as diazepam and midazolam undergo large increases in pharmacokinetic Vd, explained by the propensity of the drug to be taken up into the excess adipose tissue (Abernethy and Greenblatt, 1982). Based on Eq. (4), this leads to proportional prolongation of elimination half-life. Another circumstance in which body composition changes is in old age. The aging process is associated with a reduction in lean body mass, with a concurrent increase in adipose tissue mass, relative to total body weight (Greenblatt et al, 1982b). This will occur in elderly individuals even though they maintain "normal" body weight, exercise regularly, and eat what could be considered a reasonable diet. These age-related alterations in body habitus, although not nearly as obvious as those observed in morbid obesity, nonetheless can importantly influence the patterns of drug distribution. For highly lipid soluble drugs, Vd will increase as a function of age. For water soluble drugs, on the other hand, Vd may decrease with aging (Greenblatt et al, 1982a). These changes in drug distribution occur independently of any changes that may also take place in drug clearance. Although changes in drug distribution as such do not alter steady-state concentration during multiple dosage, distribution may importantly alter the pharmacodynamic profile of drugs following single doses. In this way, drug distribution may influence drug effects in the elderly, independent of changes in clearance (See below).

Drug Distribution and Pharmacodynamic Action

It is often assumed that the duration of a drug's pharmacodynamic action following single doses parallels its elimination half-life (Greenblatt, 1985). That is, a drug with a long elimination half-life will have a long duration of action, whereas a short half-life drug will have a short duration of action. This assumption is another that is unsupported by experimental evidence. The extent of drug distribution rather than its elimination half-life may actually be the most important determinant of its duration of action following single doses, particularly when given by the intravenous route. For a drug whose in vivo behavior is consistent with a two-compartment model, elimination half-life is calculated only after distribution is complete. Therefore the half-life as such provides no information on the rate or extent of drug distribution. For highly lipophilic drugs such as diazepam, plasma concentrations may fall rapidly and precipitously in the initial phase of drug distribution, usually lasting for a few hours after intravenous drug administration (Fig. 1). Diazepam

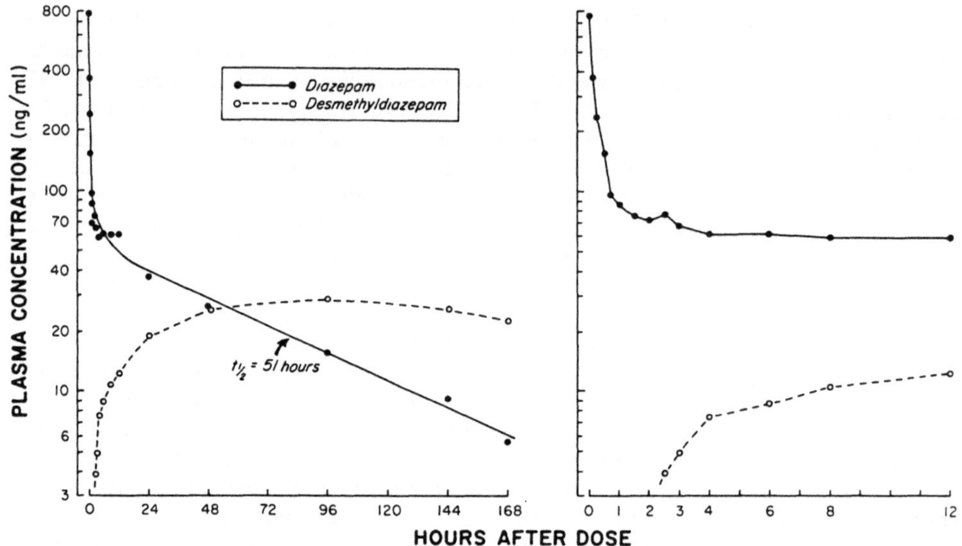

Fig.1

Plasma concentrations of diazepam and its major metabolite, desmethyldiazepam, in healthy volunteer subject following a single 10-mg intravenous dose of diazepam. Concentrations were measured at frequent intervals during 7 days (168 hours) after the dose. Left: Kinetic analysis of diazepam during the entire 7-day period demonstrates the slow rate of elimination after distribution is complete. Right: Magnification of the initial 12 hour period after dosage shows the extensive early fall in plasma diazepam concentrations due to distribution.

concentrations may fall by tenfold or more in the first few hours after a single intravenous dose. Thereafter, after distribution equilibrium has been attained, the rate of disappearance from plasma is greatly slowed. The slow rate of diazepam elimination (that is, the long elimination half-life) observed in the post-distributive phase is due partly to its low metabolic clearance, and partly to its very large Vd, as predicted by Eq. (4). Furthermore, the duration of action of a single therapeutic dose of diazepam given intravenously is relatively short, lasting anywhere from a few minutes to a few hours. It is this rapid and extensive phase of drug distribution that accounts for the rapid termination of diazepam's action following single intravenous doses. Even though the drug's elimination half-life is long, and it may be detected in plasma and in target organs for many days or even weeks after a single dose, the pharmacodynamic action is terminated much more rapidly by the extensive decline in plasma concentrations in the initial distribution phase. The importance of distribution in terminating the pharmacodynamic action of lipophilic drugs has been demonstrated in both experimental and clinical studies (Arendt et al, 1983; Greenblatt, 1985).

Drug Distribution and Clinical Effects in the Elderly

Important changes in the pharmacokinetics of drug distribution may occur in association with the aging process. Since distribution may be a major determinant of drug pharmacodynamics after single doses, the relation of drug distribution to drug sensitivity in the elderly is a research area of both basic and clinical importance.

Acknowledgements

This work was supported in part by Grants MH-34223 and AG-00106 from the United States Public Health Service.

References

Abernethy, D. R., Greenblatt, D. J.: Pharmacokinetics of drugs in obesity. Clin. Pharmacokin. 7, 108–124, 1982.

Arendt, R. M., Greenblatt, D. J., deJong, R. H., Bonin, J. D., Abernethy, D. R., Ehrenberg, B. L., Giles, H. G., Sellers, E. M., Shader, R. I.: In vitro correlates of benzodiazepine cerebrospinal fluid uptake, pharmacodynamic action, and peripheral distribution. J. Pharmacol. Exp. Ther. 227, 95–106, 1983.

Chiou, W. L.: Potential effect of early blood sampling schedule on calculated pharmacokinetic parameters of drugs after intravenous administration. J. Pharm. Sci. 69, 867–869, 1980.

Chiou, W. L., Lam, G., Chen, M.-L., Lee, M. G.: Instantaneous input hypothesis in pharmacokinetic studies. J. Pharm. Sci. 70, 1037–1039, 1981.

Friedman, H., Abernethy, D. R., Greenblatt, D. J., Shader, R. I.: The pharmacokinetics of diazepam and desmethyldiazepam in rat brain and plasma. Psychopharmacology (in press, 1985c).

Friedman, H., Ochs, H. R., Greenblatt, D. J., Shader, R. I.: Tissue distribution of diazepam and its metabolite desmethyldiazepam: a human autopsy study. J. Clin. Pharmacol. (in press, 1985a).

Friedman, H. L., Scavone, J. M., Greenblatt, D. J., Shader, R. I.: Effect of age and body composition on benzodiazepine distribution in rats. Pharmacologist 27, 207, 1985b.

Greenblatt, D. J.: Elimination half-life of drugs: value and limitations. Ann. Rev. Med. 36, 421–427, 1985.

Greenblatt, D. J., Divoll, M., Abernethy, D. R., Shader, R. I.: Physiologic changes in old age: relation to altered drug disposition. J. Am. Geriatr. Soc. 30 (November supplement), S6–S10, 1982b.

Greenblatt, D. J., Sellers, E. M., Shader, R. I.: Drug disposition in old age. N. Engl. J. Med. 306, 1081–1088, 1982a.

Greenblatt, D. J., Koch-Weser, J.: Clinical pharmacokinetics. N. Engl. J. Med. 293, 702–705, 964–970, 1975.

Greenblatt, D. J., Shader, R. I.: Pharmacokinetics in Clinical Practice. Philadelphia, W. B. Saunders, 1985.

Greenblatt, D. J., Allen, M. D., Harmatz, J. S., Shader, R. I.: Diazepam disposition determinants. Clin. Pharmacol. Ther. 27, 301–312, 1980.

Greenblatt, D. J., Arendt, R. M.: Lipid solubility and brain uptake of benzodiazepines. Pharmacologist 27, 207, 1985.

Greenblatt, D. J., Matlis, R., Scavone, J. M., Blyden, G. T., Harmatz, J. S., Shader, R. I.: Oxaprozin pharmacokinetics in the elderly. Brit. J. Clin. Pharmacol. 19, 373–378, 1985.

Greenblatt, D. M., Abernethy, D. R., Matlis, R., Harmatz, J. S., Shader, R. I.: Absorption and disposition of ibuprofen in the elderly. Arth. Rheum. 27, 1066–1069, 1984.

Greenblatt, D. J., Abernethy, D. R., Divoll, M.: Is volume of distribution at steady-state a meaningful kinetic variable? J. Clin. Pharmacol. 23, 391–400, 1983a.

Greenblatt, D. J., Arendt, R. M., Abernethy, D. R., Giles, H. G., Sellers, E. M., Shader, R. I.: In vitro quantitation of benzodiazepine lipophilicity: relation to in vivo distribution. Brit. J. Anaesthes. 55, 985–989, 1983b.

Klotz, U.: Pathophysiological and disease-induced changes in drug distribution volume: pharmacokinetic implications. Clin. Pharmacokinet. 1, 204–218, 1976.

Niazi, S.: Errors involved in instantaneous intravascular input assumptions. J. Pharm. Sci. 65, 750–752, 1976.

Ochs, H. R., Greenblatt, D. J., Abernethy, D. R., Arendt, R. M., Gerloff, J., Eichelkraut, W., Hahn, N.: Cerebrospinal fluid uptake and peripheral distribution of centrally acting drugs: relation to lipid solubility. J. Pharm. Pharmacol. 37, 428–431, 1985.

Ritschel, W. A., Hammer, G. V.: Prediction of the volume of distribution from in vitro data and use for estimating the absolute extent of absorption. Int. J. Clin. Pharmacol. Ther. Toxicol. 18, 298–316, 1980.

Sjöqvist, F., Alván, G.: Aging and drug disposition: Metabolism. J. Chronic. Dis 36, 31–37, 1983.

Schmucker, D. L.: Aging and drug disposition: an update. Pharmacol. Rev. 37, 133–148, 1985.

Verbeeck, R. K., Blackburn, J. L., Loewen, G. R.: Clinical pharmacokinetics of non-steroidal anti-inflammatory drugs. Clin. Pharmacokin. 8, 297–331, 1983.

Vestal, R. E.; Wood, A. J. J., Shand, D. G.: Reduced β-adrenoceptor sensitivity in the elderly. Clin. Pharmacol. Ther. 26, 181–186, 1979.

Vestal, R. E.: Pharmacology and aging. J. Am. Geriatr. Soc. 30, 191–200, 1982.

Einfluß des Alters auf die hepatische Elimination von Koffein, Hexobarbital und Lidocain in einem internistischen Patientenkollektiv

R. Joeres, H. Heusler, G. Hofstetter, D. Brachtel, H. Gallenkamp, H. Reuß, H. Klinker, J. Epping, E. Richter
Medizinische Universitätsklinik, D-8700 Würzburg

W. Zilly
Hartwaldklinik, D-8788 Bad Brückenau

Summary

The liver, like other organs, undergoes age dependent atrophy. Physiological functions are not critically diminished, whereas oxidative drug metabolism is impaired for many substrates. This may be the reason for a higher incidence of adverse drug reactions in the elderly. We studied the influence of age on the hepatic elimination of two low clearance model-substrates of the oxidative metabolism, hexobarbital (cytochrome P 450) and caffeine (cytochrome P 448), and of lidocaine, a high clearance drug, in patients without liver disease and after exclusion of interfering factors (smoking, inducing drugs and oral contraceptives). Plasma concentrations of the three drugs were determined by gaschromatography and pharmacokinetic parameters were calculated from a one compartment open model (caffeine, hexobarbital) or in steady state (lidocaine). Caffeine clearance decreased significantly with age (15—88 years) with corresponding changes in halflife, whereas volume of distribution was not influenced (Clearance (ml/min) = 94.16 − 0.56 x years, r = 0.52, n = 61). Less pronounced, but also significant changes for the 12 h plasma-concentration of hexobarbital and the lidocaine clearance could be demonstrated. However, the effect of liver disease completely overrules the influence of age on caffeine and hexobarbital elimination and the same holds true for pump failure of the heart in the case of lidocaine. We conclude, that in comparison with age dependent impairment of oxidative liver metabolism other clinical conditions are of greater importance for the adjustment of a dosage regimen in pharmacotherapy of the elderly. Nevertheless appropriate dose reduction can be recommended in general in old age.

Zusammenfassung

In einem lebergesunden Patientenkollektiv findet sich nach Ausschluß von Interaktionen (Rauchen, orale Kontrazeptiva und induzierende Begleitmedikation) eine altersabhänge Abnahme der hepatischen Elimination von Koffein, Hexobarbital und Lidocain. Wesentlich stärkere und den Einfluß des Alters überdeckende Veränderungen finden sich jedoch bei Lebererkrankungen wie Hepatitis und Leberzirrhose.

Grundsätzlich sollte jedoch der Verminderung des oxydativen Arzneimittelmetabolismus im Alter durch eine Dosisanpassung Rechnung getragen werden.

Wie viele andere Organe unterliegt die Leber einer Altersinvolution. Physiologische Stoffwechselleistungen sind dabei nicht erkennbar eingeschränkt (Blutgerinnung, Glukoneogenese und die Funktion des retikuloendothelialen Systems) [1—4]. Nach neueren Befunden kann vermutet werden, daß höheres Alter durch metabolisch veränderte Zusammensetzung der Galle einen Risikofaktor für die Gallensteinbildung darstellt [5]. Es ist eine bekannte klinische Tatsache, daß die Leber des älteren Menschen eine geringere Regenerationsfähigkeit besitzt, und Hepatitiserkrankungen schwerer und langwieriger verlaufen [6].
In der Altersklasse, die am häufigsten einer Pharmakotherapie bedarf und in der die meisten Nebenwirkungen auftreten, ließ sich für viele Arzneimittel und klassische quantitative Leberfunktionsproben eine Einschränkung der hepatischen Stoffwechselleistung nachweisen [7—9].
Im folgenden wird der Einfluß des Alters in einem lebergesunden Patientenkollektiv auf die fast ausschließliche hepatische Elimination der low-clearance-Substanzen Koffein [10] und Hexobarbital [11] und der high-clearance-Substanz Lidocain [12] dargestellt.
Methodik: Die Konzentrationsbestimmung von Koffein, Lidocain und Hexobarbital im Plasma erfolgten nach Flüssigextraktionen im definierten pH-Bereich durch Kapillargaschromatographie [13, 14].
Die Koffein- und Hexobarbitalclearances wurden — soweit vollständige Plasmakonzentrationsverlaufskurven vorhanden sind — als D/AUC berechnet. Bei einem Teil der Patienten, in denen während der Resorptionsphase keine Meßwerte zur Verfügung standen, wurden die Clearances aus dem loglinearen Anteil der Plasmakonzentrationskurve nach der Forml $V_D \times Ln2/t_{1/2}$ errechnet. Die Lidocain-Clearance bei den Patienten mit Myocardinfakt wurde aus der in der Zeiteinheit infundierten Dosis und den steady-state-Plasmakonzentrationen errechnet (CL = D (ug/min)/C (ug/ml)).
Ergebnisse: Pharmakokinetische Parameter des Koffein als relativ reines Cytochrom P 448-Substrat wurden bei 61 Patienten und gesunden Probanden gemessen. Ausgeschlossen waren Patienten mit Lebererkrankungen und sonstigen schweren Krankheitsbildern und Personen, die enzyminduzierenden oder inhibierenden Einflüssen ausgesetzt waren (Rauchen, orale Kontrazeptiva, Begleitmedikation wie Antiepileptika und Cimetidin). Tabelle I zeigt die Abnahme der Koffeinclearance mit zunehmendem Alter und eine entsprechende Zunahme der Eliminationshalbwertzeit. Das Verteilungsvolumen zeigte keine signifikanten Veränderungen mit dem Alter, insbesondere bleibt das relative Verteilungsvolumen mit 0,45 l/kg KG über den gesamten Altersbereich konstant. Die individuellen Meßwerte der Koffeinclearance sind in Abb. 1 gegen das Alter aufgetragen. Hiernach ergibt sich bei einer erheblichen Streuung eine signifikante negative Korrelation zwischen beiden Größen im Gegensatz zu einer früheren Publikation [10], in der aber eine wesentlich geringere Anzahl von Probanden zur Verfügung stand. Frauen weisen nach unseren Ergebnissen eine gering niedrigere Koffeinclearance als Männer auf; dieser Unterschied ist aber wohl Folge des in gleichem Maße niedrigeren Körpergewichts bei Frauen, denn nach entsprechender Korrektur findet sich kein Einfluß des Geschlechtes auf die Koffeinclearance mehr. Es sei auch darauf hingewiesen, daß die altersabhängige Abnahme der Koffeinclearance nicht etwa durch eine ebenfalls altersabhängige Gewichtsabnahme bedingt ist, da sich in unserem Kollektiv kein derartiger Zusammenhang nachweisen läßt.

Tabelle 1 Pharmakokinetische Parameter des Koffein bei 61 lebergesunden Patienten und gesunden Probanden im Alter von 15—88 Jahren

Alter	♀ : ♂	Cl (ml/min)	t 1/2 (min)	Vd (l)
28 ± 8 (15 – 39) n = 17	10 : 7	80 ± 23	292 ± 104	32 ± 9
56 ± 8 (40 – 69) n = 17	5 : 12	63 ± 20	376 ± 147	30 ± 6
76 ± 6 (70 – 88) n = 27	11 : 16	51 ± 18	431 ± 259	28 ± 10

Mittelwerte ± Standardabweichung

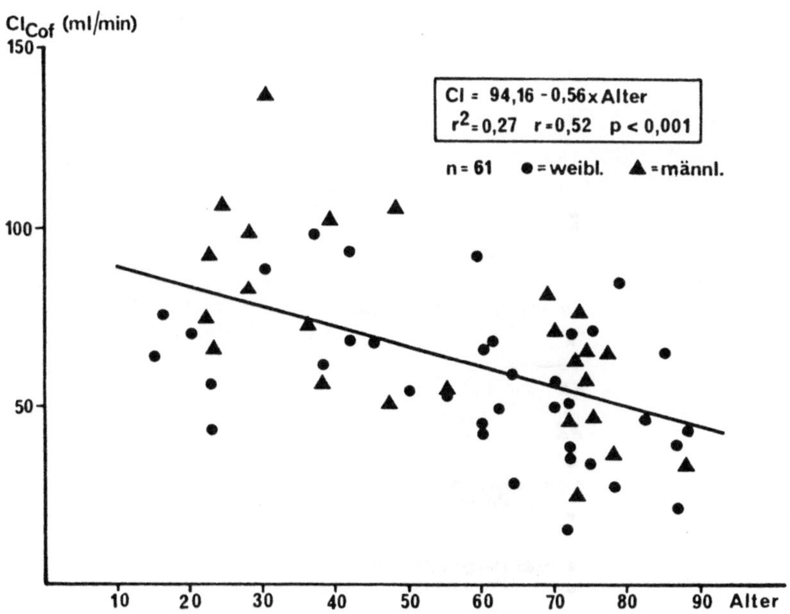

Abb. 1

Beziehung zwischen Koffeinclearance und Alter bei 61 Patienten (ausgeschlossen waren Leberkranke und der Einfluß von Enzyminduktoren und Inhibitoren).

Für Hexobarbital, das als Cytochrom P 450-Substrat gilt und dessen Elimination durch Rauchen nicht beeinflußt wird, findet sich ebenfalls eine Verminderung der Clearance im Alter. Dementsprechend liegen die 12-Stunden-Plasmakonzentrationen nach oraler Gabe von 250 mg Hexobarbital im Mittel bei Lebergesunden über 50 Jahren signifikant höher als bei jüngeren Patienten (Abb. 2). Einschränkend muß aber gesagt werden, daß drei der vier ältesten Patienten — in der Abb. markiert — durchaus in einem Bereich liegen, der auch bei Jüngeren vorgefunden wird. Insgesamt gibt es große Überschneidungen in beiden Altersgruppen, so daß im Einzelfall eine Vorhersage des Alterseinflusses nicht möglich ist.

Ähnliche Resultate ergibt die Lidocainclearance bei Patienten mit akutem Myokardinfarkt ohne Leber-, Nieren- oder Herzinsuffizienz (Abb. 3). Lidocain, das überwiegend N-deethyliert wird, wird bei diesen Patienten als Antiarrhythmikum eingesetzt. Bei insgesamt großer Streuung der Werte liegt bei Älteren die Lidocainclearance, wenn auch gering, so doch statistisch signifikant niedriger als bei den Patienten unter 65 Jahren.

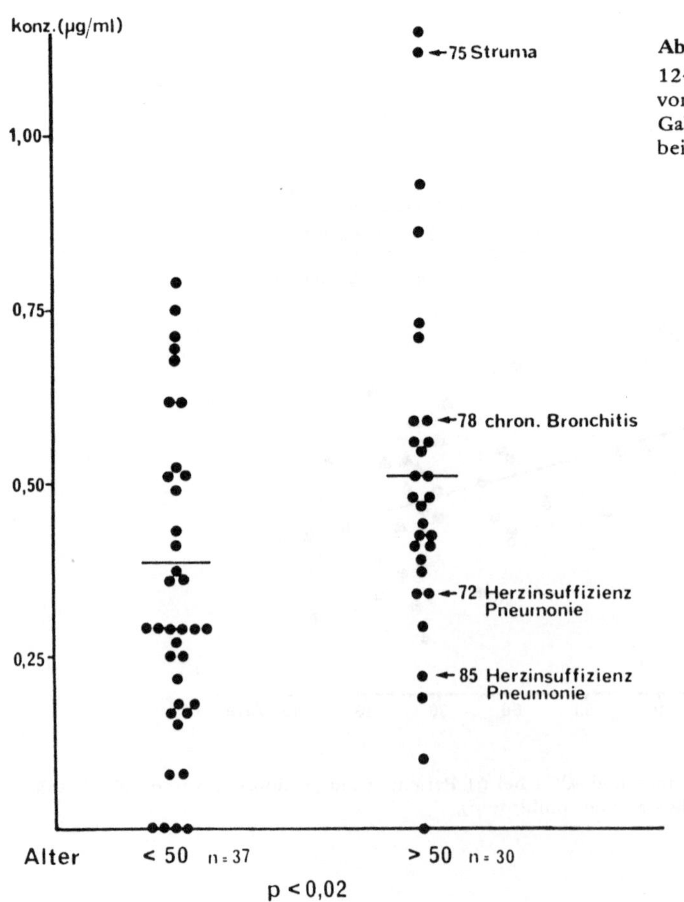

Abb. 2

12-Stunden-Plasmakonzentration von Hexorbartibal nach oraler Gabe von 250 mg Hexobarbital bei 67 lebergesunden Patienten.

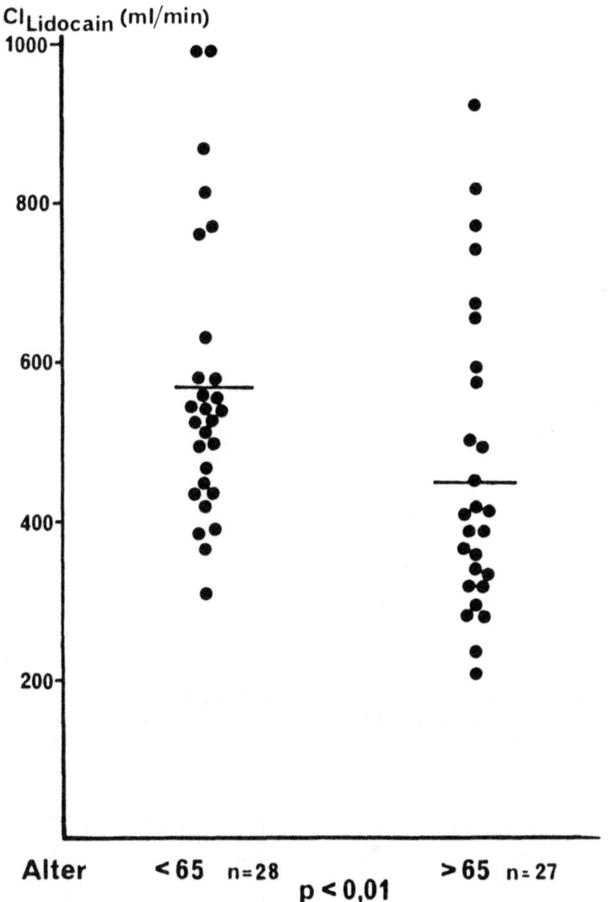

Abb. 3
Lidocainclearance bei 55 Patienten mit akutem Myocardinfarkt (keine Leber-, Nieren- oder Herzinsuffizienz).

Bei allen drei verwendeten Modellsubstraten ergibt sich nach unseren Befunden bei strenger Auswahl der Probanden eine Abnahme der Elimination mit dem Alter. Der klinische Stellenwert dieser Beobachtung wird aber durch die Tatsache relativiert, daß andere, insbesondere krankheitsbedingte Änderungen der Leberfunktion einen wesentlichen größen Einfluß besitzen. Untersucht man die Lidocainclearance in einem nicht selektierten Kollektiv, so läßt sich kein Einfluß des Alters mehr nachweisen. Dies gilt auch für Hexobarbital und Koffein, wenn zusätzlich Lebererkrankungen vorliegen (Abb. 4, 5). Bei der akuten Hepatitis und insbesondere bei Patienten mit Leberzirrhose findet sich eine Einschränkung des Metabolismus, die weit über den Einfluß des Alters hinausgeht und diesen auch nicht mehr nachweisbar werden läßt.

Die dargestellten Ergebnisse legen, soweit eine Verallgemeinerung möglich ist, den Schluß nahe, daß die Stoffwechselleistung der Leber im Alter abnimmt, ohne daß bei Fehlen sonstiger Erkrankungen ein kritischer Wert erreicht würde. Erhöhte Belastungen — hierzu zählt auch eine Pharmakotherapie — und Begleiterkrankungen dagegen schränken die

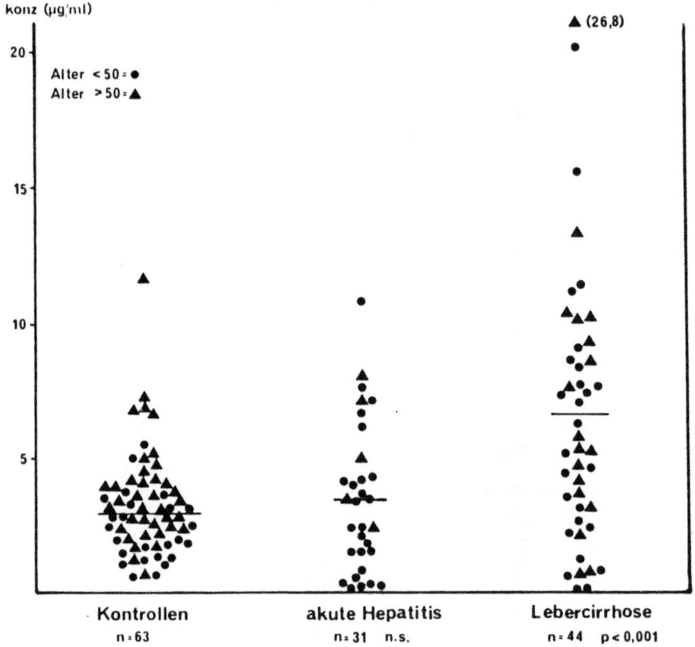

Abb. 4

12-Stunden-Plasmakonzentrationen nach oraler Gabe von 366 mg Koffein bei Kontrollen (n = 63), Patienten mit akuter Hepatitis (n = 31) und Leberzirrhose (n = 44).

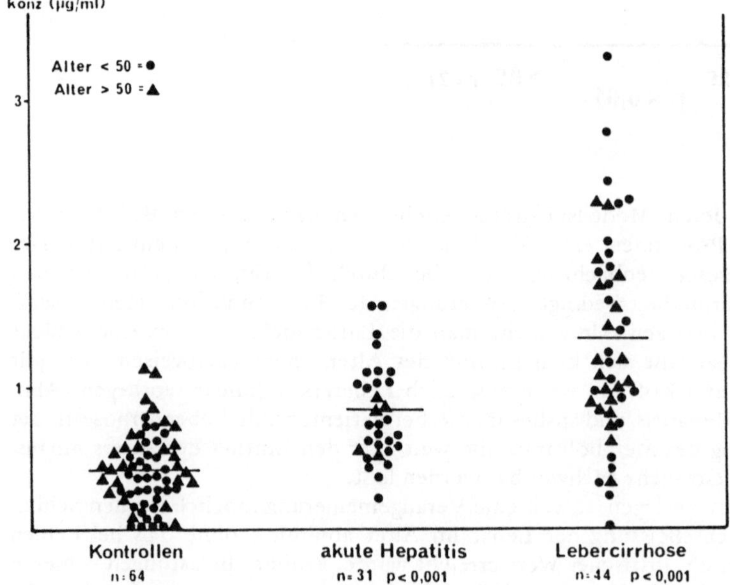

Abb. 5

12-Stunden-Plasmakonzentrationen nach oraler Gabe von 250 mg Hexobarbital bei Kontrollen (n = 64), Patienten mit akuter Hepatits (n = 31) und Leberzirrhose (n = 44).

Leberfunktion wesentlich stärker ein und erfordern entsprechende therapeutische Konsequenzen. In jedem Fall erscheint es geraten, eine medikamentöse Therapie auf ein sinnvolles Mindestmaß zu beschränken.
Frl. U. Müller und Frl. D. Schirmer danken wir für die Durchführung der Laboranalysen und Frau K. Köhler für die Anfertigung des Manuskripts.
Mit Unterstützung durch die DFG.

Literatur

[1] *Kühn, H. A., Wernze, H.:* Klinische Hepatologie, Thieme-Verlag, Stuttgart (1979)

[2] *Kitani,* (Ed.): Liver and aging. Elsevier Biomedical, Amsterdam (1982)

[3] *Platt, D.* (Ed.): Liver and aging. Schattauer-Verlag, Stuttgart (1977)

[4] *James, O. F. W.:* Gastrointestinal and liver function in old age. *Lusowsky, M. S.* (Ed.): Clinics in Gastroentology, Vol. **12** (1983), Saunders, Philadelphia.

[5] *Einarsson, K., Nielsill, K., Leijd, B., Angelin, B.:* Influence of age on secretion of cholesterol and synthesis of bile acids by the liver. New Engl. J. Med., **313**, 277−282 (1985)

[6] *Kühn, H. A.:* Akute und chronische Hepatitiden im Alter. Dtsch. Ztschr. f. Verdauungs- und Stoffwechselkrankheiten, **32**, 49−54 (1972)

[7] *Vesell, E. S.:* Der Einfluß von Wirtsfaktoren auf die Wirkung von Medikamenten II. Alter Internist, **22**, 99−105 (1981)

[8] *Shand, D. G.:* Biological determinants of altered pharmakokinetics in the elderly. Gerontology, **28**, Supll. 1, 8−17 (1982)

[9] *Greenblatt, D. J., Sellers, E. M., Shader, R. J.:* Drug disposition in old age. New Engl. J. Med., **306**, 1081−1088 (1982)

[10] *Blanchard, J., Sawers, S. J. A.:* Comparative pharmakokinetics of caffein in young and elderly man. J. Pharmacokinetics and Biopharm., **11**, 109−126 (1983)

[11] *Vermeulen, N. P. E., Rietveld, C. T., Breimer, D. D.:* Disposition of hexobarbitone in healthy man: Kinetics of parent drug and metabolites following oral administration. Brit. J. Clin. Pharmacol., **15**, 459−464 (1983)

[12] *Lelorier, J., Grenon, D., Latour, Y., Caille, G., Dumont, G., Brosseau, A., Solignac, A.:* Pharmacokinetics of Lidocain after prolonged intravenous infusion in uncomplicated myocardial infarction. Ann. Int. Med., **87**, 700−702 (1977)

[13] *Heusler, H., Richter, E.:* Quantitative Bestimmung von Koffein in biologischen Flüssigkeiten mit Hilfe der Gaschromatographie und N-selektiver Detektion. In: Rietbrook, N. et al. (Hrsg.), Theophyllin and other methylxanthines. Methods in clinical pharmacology no. 3, Vieweg u. Sohn, Braunschweig, Wiesbaden (1981)

[14] *Heusler, H.:* Quantitative analysis of common anaesthetic agents. J. Chromatography, **340**, 273− 319 (1985)

Drug Evaluation in the Elderly

I. H. Stevenson
Department of Pharmacology and Clinical Pharmacology, Ninewells Hospital and Medical School, Dundee, DD1 9SY, Scotland

Summary

This paper surveys the variety of methods used within the group in Dundee investigating drug response in the elderly. A broad approch has been used ranging from epidemiological studies on problems of drug use in old people to intensive laboratory evaluation of pharmacokinetics or pharmacodynamics following single and multiple dose treatment.
The problems of evaluating new drugs in the elderly are reviewed along with some of the measures which are being taken to improve the present situation.

In the U.K. and many other countries drug use is disproportionately high in the older age groups and, moreover, the number of prescriptions is increasing more rapidly than is the number of old people in the country [1]. The age-related increase in rate of adverse reaction to some drugs is well documented and, probably more so than any other factor, the adverse event problem — highlighted by the withdrawal of benoxaprofen in 1982 — has been responsible for the marked interest in geriatric clinical pharmacology over the last ten years [2]. This has resulted in the elucidation of some of the underlying mechanisms, principally alterations in pharmacokinetics or pharmacodynamics or impairment of physiological homeostasis as people age.
In view of the considerable medical and economic importance of the prescribing of drugs for the elderly there is clearly still a great need for further research in order to allow in older patients as safe and effective a use of existing drugs as possible and to contribute to the development of appropriate new medicines for this age group.
It is the objective of this paper to review the various approaches used in Dundee over a period of years largely under the direction of the late Professor James Crooks, in the investigation of age-related differences in drug use, efficacy and fate and to examine the problems of new drug evaluation in the elderly.

Approaches to Study of Drugs in the Elderly

Table I summarises the various approaches which have been used in Dundee over the last fifteen years. These can be broadly classified as studies in volunteers, in hospital inpatients or patients attending hospital outpatient or general practice clinics and community-based studies in elderly patients carried out within their homes. The studies carried out may be further sub-grouped into epidemiological or laboratory-based, the latter group including both single and multiple-dose pharmacokinetic and pharmacodynamic investigations.

Table I Approaches used in studying drugs in the elderly

A. Patient Studies

1. Epidemiology of drug use
2. Epidemiological studies on drug efficacy
3. Single dose pharmacodynamic studies
4. Single dose pharmacokinetic studies
5. Multiple dose pharmacodynamic studies
6. Multiple dose pharmacokinetic studies.

B. Volunteer Studies

1. Single dose pharmacokinetic studies
2. Single dose pharmacodynamic studies

C. Community-Based Studies

1. Assessment of drug effect in relation to plasma concentration.

Epidemiology of Drug Use — Hypnotics

The "Crooks" system of hospital drug recording was introduced in North-East Scotland in 1965 [3] and has since been widely adopted. More recently different methodology has been developed in Dundee to provide data on prescribing in general practice [4]. The system was used to examine the prescribing of hypnotics in patients of 65 years or over and clearly showed that benzodiazepines as expected, were the most frequently prescribed group (64.6 % of all prescriptions) followed by barbiturates (24.6 %) with all others accounting for only 10.8 %. Only 2 benzodiazepines were used to any extent — nitrazepam and flurazepam, the former accounting for approximately 5 times the prescriptions of the latter. The system permitted analysis of dose and showed, for example, that of the doses of nitrazepam prescribed for the over 65's only 42 % were 5 mg (maximum dose) or lower with 32 % being greater than 5 mg and a further 26 % unknown. This example therefore serves to illustrate the usefulness of such a system in documenting patterns of drug use and of drug dose in elderly patients.

Epidemiological Studies on Drug Efficacy — Warfarin

Studies by O'Malley et al. [5] using inpatient anticoagulant records along with information on anticoagulant dose showed that the quality of anticoagulant control was rather poor but, if anything, tended to improve with age of patient. Moreover, the study indicated a possible increase in sensitivity to the anticoagulant warfarin in elderly patients since, despite receiving lower doses, they showed a significantly increased anticoagulant effect (in terms of reduction in Thrombotest). This was subsequently confirmed in a further prospective survey [6] carried out in the anticoagulant clinic.

Single Dose Pharmacodynamic Studies in Patients — Warfarin, Benoxaprofen

These studies by Shepherd et al. [7] were undertaken to determine whether the apparent age-related increase in sensitivity to warfarin could be demonstrated in man in a single

50

dose study under precisely defined conditions. Prothrombin complex activity was significantly lower (i. e. greater suppression of synthesis) at virtually all time points over a 120 h study period despite the elderly patients receiving lower doses. To assess the relative sensitivity of clotting factor synthesis to warfarin in the two age groups, the rate of synthesis of clotting factors was plotted against the logarithm of plasma warfarin concentration. At the same plasma warfarin concentration the geriatric group showed a much greater degree of inhibition of Vitamin K-dependent factor synthesis than did the young group.

Single Dose Pharmacokinetic Studies in Patients — Warfarin, Benoxaprofen

In investigating the possible mechanism of the age-related increase in sensitivity to warfarin, studies were carried out to compare the single dose pharmacokinetics of the drug in the two age groups [7]. Although the mean half-life of warfarin was longer and the plasma clearance slightly lower in the elderly patients, the differences between the means were not statistically significant. There was no difference between the apparent volumes of distribution or between the extent of warfarin plasma protein binding in the two age groups.

In a more recent study [8] in elderly arthritic outpatients (i. e. relatively healthy elderly patients living at home) the elimination half life of benoxaprofen (47.6 h) was found to be longer than that value reported for healthy young subjects (25.7 h) but considerably lower than that reported in two hospital inpatient studies (101 and 111 hours). This draws attention to the heterogeneity of the elderly as a group and to the need to define fully the population under study. The results for benoxaprofen would suggest that, based on half-life data, the elimination of the drug is less influenced by age per se than by hospitalisation and the factors associated with this, principally severity of illness.

Multiple Dose Pharmacokinetic Studies in Patients — Propranolol

Propanolol is widely used in the management of hyperthyroid patients of all ages and its single dose pharmacokinetics has been investigated in a number of studies. The purpose of the study by Feely et al [9] was to determine if ageing influenced the plasma propanolol steady state concentations achieved during the treatment of hyperthyroid patients. An age correlation was found with plasma propanolol steady state levels increasing very strikingly with age. This correlation held irrespective of smoking status and thyroid function.

Multiple Dose Pharmacodynamic Studies in Patients — Propanolol

The Feely study [9] also investigated the degree of β-adrenoceptor blockade (assessed from the reduction in exercise tachycardia) and examined the relationship between degree of blockade (related to plasma propranolol steady state level) and age of the patient. In this case a significant negative correlation was found indicating that, although higher plasma propranolol steady state levels are found in elderly patients there is a concomitant reduction in the sensitivity to propranolol with ageing.

Single Dose Pharmacokinetic Studies in Volunteers — Antipyrine, Zimelidine

The study by O'Malley et al [10] on antipyrine was the first to indicate an impariment of drug metabolism as people age. Similar results have since been reported with a great many drugs. Antipyrine has also been used in attempts to elucidate whether or not the induction response is influenced by ageing [11]. The indications from this and other studies is that there may be a reduction in the extent of induction in older subjects although studies to date suffer from the defect that induction is only assessed at one time point and if, as is known to occur in old animals, the induction response is merely slower it could well be missed or under-estimated.

Pharmacokinetic studies on the antidepressant zimelidine [12] showed a gross difference between young and elderly in the single dose plasma concentration versus time profiles. The AUC for zimelidine in the elderly was some 3 1/2 times that in the young with the elimination half lives of zimelidine and its metabolite norzimelidine being prolonged in the older group. The data were interpreted as a small reduction in the rate of hepatic biotransformation of zimelidine in the elderly combined with a more extensive increase in total bioavailability.

Single Dose Pharmacodynamic Studies in Volunteers — Chlormethiazole

Considerable effort has been expended in the investigation of immediate and hangover effects of hypnotics in elderly and young healthy volunteers. Effects were assessed using body sway, choice reaction time and critical flicker fusion threshold. The studies on chlormethiazole [13] indicated that the elderly were more sensitive than the young to equal doses of the drug and this difference was not due to higher plasma levels of chlormethiazole occurring in the older group. The differences detected were short-lived and may indicate a reduction in the ability of the ageing brain to adapt to the drugs effect although other possible explanations exist.

Determination of Drug Effect in Relation to Plasma Concentration — A Study on Benzodiazepines Carried Out in Elderly Patients at Home

The increased effect of single doses of benzodiazepines in the elderly (for example — the exaggerated effects on body sway) has been demonstrated in other studies in this department [13] and, with the information from epidemiological surveys on benzodiazepine use in the elderly a particular problem with benzodiazepines in the elderly at home might have been predicted. In the study by Swift et al [14] a significant proportion of elderly patients had been receiving nitrazepam for in excess of 10 years. Measurement of the plasma concentration of nitrazepam in the patients under study revealed a good correlation with dose indicating good compliance within the patient population. In some of the elderly subjects studied, very high plasma concentrations of nitrazepam were found. In assessing the nitrazepam response in this group, in terms of effect on body sway, it was surprising to find that no correlation existed between sway and nitrazepam plasma concentration and the findings suggest the development of some degree of tolerance to the side effects of nitrazepam in elderly patients.

New Drug Evaluation in the Elderly

As a result of adverse drug events in the elderly, much thought has been given by regulatory authorities to the problem of the proper evaluation and use of drugs in this age group. The Committee on Safety of Medicines, for example, has recommended [1] that, where relevant, Drug Data Sheets should include a statement of advice on the use and effect of individual drugs in the elderly — covering dose, dose intervals and possible side effects. Where no information is available relating to the elderly it is thought that it may be helpful to say so.

It has also recommended that "where appropriate" drugs should be evaluated in elderly subjects as part of an application for a product licence. The appropriateness would depend on such as factors as expected extent of use of the drug in the elderly, therapeutic index and likely changes in pharmacokinetics and pharmacodynamics with age.

Table II lists the types of drugs which are possibly likely to produce special problems in the elderly and which might be considered as appropriate for full evaluation in the elderly. While some of the problems are readily recognised and dealt with — e. g. the need to assess the effects of impaired renal excretion for renally excreted drugs, the prospect of evaluating all psychoactive drugs in the elderly is daunting.

Even accepting the appropriateness of selection of particular drugs for evaluation in the elderly a number of further problems arise (Table III). The recruitment of elderly subjects, whether volunteers or patients is difficult and time consuming and availability of elderly subjects is likely to be a limiting factor in many cases. The elderly are also a very heterogeneous group ranging from "fit old folk" to the debilitated elderly and even within subgroups of the elderly population standard deviation from the mean for results tends to be higher than that in younger groups and may lead to statistical difficulties in comparing results.

Table II Drugs liable to produce special problems in the Elderly

<table>
<tr><td>

1. Drugs intended for widespread use in elderly populations
2. Drugs with a steep dose-response curve and low therapeutic ratio — particularly if:
    (a)   eliminated by renal mechanisms
    (b)   undergoes first-pass extraction.
3. Psychoactive drugs
4. Drugs whose effects are likely to be modified by homeostatic mechanisms.

</td></tr>
</table>

Table III Drug evaluation in the elderly

<table>
<tr><td>

Difficulties Encountered

1. Relevance of studies in healthy elderly volunteers.
2. Recruitment problems.
3. Elderly group heterogeneous, ranging from "fit old folk" to the debilitated elderly.
4. Standard deviation of results high — statistical difficulties.
5. Presence of disease.
6. Sex differences may complicate studies.

</td></tr>
</table>

One further major problem is that of the relevance of using healthy elderly subjects for the evaluation of drugs ultimately intended for the sick elderly. The approach of using elderly patients for whom a drug is intended e.g. elderly hypertensives, elderly diabetics etc. is sensible but is unlikely to provide the complete answer. There is considerable evidence that drug problems in the elderly occur particularly in the debilitated or very sick elderly patient often receiving chronic multiple drug therapy and a trial evaluation of new drugs under such circumstances would not be possible. While adoption of some of the measures outlined are likely to reduce drug problems occurring in the elderly, they are unlikely to eliminate them.

References

[1] CSM Update — Drugs and the Elderly, **290**, 1345 (1985).
[2] *Friedel, R. O.:* Introduction — Gerontology 28 (Suppl. 1): 5—7 (1982)
[3] *Crooks, J.:* Br. J. clin. Pharmac., **16**, 351—357 (1983)
[4] *Hamley, J. G., Brown, S. V., Crooks, J., Knox, J. D., Murdoch, J. C., Patterson, A. W.* and 20 Tayside General Practitioners: J. Roy. Coll. Gen. Pract., **31**, 654—660 (1981)
[5[*O'Malley, K., Stevenson, I. H., Ward, C. A., Wood, A. J. J., Crooks, J.:* Br. J. clin. Pharmac., **4**, 309—314 (1977)
[6] *Shepherd, A. M. M., Christopher, L. J., Stevenson, I. H., Henney, C. R., Brown, Y.:* Postgrad. Med. J., **54**, 784—788 (1978)
[7] *Shepherd, A. M. M., Hewick, D. S., Moreland, T. A., Stevenson, I. H.:* Br. J. clin. Pharmac. **4**, 315—320 (1977).
[8] *Stevenson, I. H., Hosie, J.:* Proceedings of the Symposium on Pharmacology and Therapeutics in the Elderly, Dublin 1985. Elsevier (in press.)
[9] *Feely, J., Stevenson, I. H.:* J. clin. Exptl. Gerontol., **1**, 173—184 (1979)
[10] *O'Malley, K., Crooks, J., Duke, E., Stevenson, I. H.:* Br. med. J., **3**, 607—609 (1971)
[11] *Salem, S. A. M., Rajjayabun, P., Shepherd, A. M. M., Stevenson, I. H.:* Age and Ageing **7**, 68—73 (1978)
[12] *Swift, C. G., Stevenson, I. H., Tiplady, B.:* Abstract 0573, World Conference on Clinical Pharmacology and Therapeutics (1980)
[13] *Stevenson, I. H., Hockings, N. F., Swift, C. G.:* Liver and Ageing, Ed. K. Kitani, p317—327. Elsevier (1982)
[14] *Swift, C. G., Swift, M. R., Hamley, J., Stevenson, I. H., Crooks, J.:* Age and Ageing **13**, 335—343 (1984)

Renal Elimination of Drugs in the Elderly

L. Dettli

Medizinische Klinik B, Kantonsspital, Universitätsklinik Basel, CH-4031 Basel

Summary

1. The over-all clearance, $\dot{V}$, of drugs eliminated partly by the kidneys depends linearly on the endogenous creatinine clearance, Cl. The decrease of $\dot{V}$ with decreasing values of Cl is the more pronounced the larger the fraction of the absorbed dose, f_{rN}, normally eliminated unchanged in the urine.
2. During adult life Cl decreases linearly with age by about 0.8 % per year.
3. It follows that the dosage regimen of drugs with a small therapeutic index and a high value of f_{rN} (e. g. digoxin, aminoglycosides) should be adjusted to the decreased functional capacity of the ageing kidney. A nomograph serving this purpose is described in the text.

Zusammenfassung

1. Die globale Plasma-Clearance $\dot{V}$ von Pharmaka, die teilweise renal eliminiert werden, nimmt linear mit der endogenen Kreatinin-Clearance Cl ab, und zwar umso ausgeprägter, je größer der Bruchteil f_{rN} der resorbierten Dosis ist, der normalerweise unverändert renal eliminiert wird.
2. Beim Erwachsenen nimmt Cl mit dem Alter um etwa 0.8 % pro Jahr linear ab.
3. Daraus folgt, daß das Dosierungsschema von Pharmaka, die durch einen kleinen therapeutischen Index und durch einen hohen Wert von f_{rN} charakterisiert sind, quantitativ der verminderten Funktionskapazität der alternden Niere angepaßt werden sollte. Eine dafür geeignete, einfache nomographische Methode wird im Text beschrieben.

In order to describe the characteristics of renal drug elimination in the aged patient the following three questions have to be answered:

1. How does renal drug elimination depend on renal function?
2. How does renal function depend on age?, and
3. How does renal drug elimination depend on extra-renal factors?

Renal Function and Drug Elimination

N. S. Bricker's "Intact nephron hypothesis" [2] states that with respect to excretory function the chronically impaired kidney may be considered as a kidney with a smaller than normal number of nephrons; in other words, the remaining nephrons are functionally normal ("intact"). This means the nephron reacts as a functional unit. In our context the important consequence is that glomerular filtration rate, tubular secretion and tubular reabsorption capacity decrease in parallel and linearly with the number of the remaining intact nephrons. It follows that any test of glomerular filtration rate such as the endogenous creatinine clearance, Cl, not only measures glomerular function, but characterizes simultaneously tubular secretion and reabsorption irrespective of the nature of the renal impairment and irrespective of the mechanisms (glomerular filtration, tubular secretion or absorption) involved in the renal handling of the drug. Based on these facts we developed our theory on the relationship between drug elimination and renal function [4, 5] which states that renal drug clearance, $\dot{V}_r$, is linearly related to the endogenous creatinine clearance, Cl. Mathematically this results in

$$\dot{V}_r = b \cdot Cl \tag{1}$$

Since total drug clearance, $\dot{V}$, is the sum of extrarenal drug clearance, $\dot{V}_{nr}$, and renal drug clearance $\dot{V}_r$, i. e.

$$\dot{V} = \dot{V}_{nr} + \dot{V}_r \tag{2}$$

introduction of eq. 1 into eq. 2 results in the following linear estimating equation describing the relationship between total drug clearance, $\dot{V}$, and creatinine clearance, Cl:

$$\dot{V} = \dot{V}_{nr} + b \cdot Cl \tag{3}$$

When it is assumed that $\dot{V}_{nr}$ remains uninfluenced by renal disease eq. 3 predicts that total drug clearance, $\dot{V}$, decreases linearly with creatinine clearance, Cl, until the extrarenal drug clearance, $\dot{V}_{nr}$ is reached in the anuric patient.

Since eq. 3 is too complicated for practical bed-side use the equation was normalized and standardized in such a way that the individual drug clearance of the patient, $\dot{V}$, is expressed as a fraction, P, of the standard drug clearance, $\dot{V}_N$, in the standard individual, i. e.

$$P = \dot{V}/\dot{V}_N \tag{4}$$

whereby the standard individual is defined by $Cl = Cl_N = 100$ ml/min. The individual drug clearance fraction, P, also decreases linearly with Cl until a minimum value — the minimal drug clearance fraction, $P_0 = \dot{V}_{nr}/\dot{V}_N$, is reached in the anuric patient with $Cl = 0$. When the value of P_0 of the drug and the patient's creatinine clearance, Cl, are known, the individual drug clearance fraction, P, in the patient can be stimated graphically in the following way by means of the simple nomograph depicted in Fig. 1: P_0 is plotted at the left ordinate and connected by a straight estimating line with the right upper corner of the nomograph. The point of intersection between the patient's creatinine clearance, Cl (lower abscissa), and the estimating line results in the individual drug clearance fraction, P, at the left ordinate.

When the standard half-life, $t_{1/2N}$, of the drug is known the half-life in the individual patient, $t_{1/2}$, is calculated in the following way from the value of P:

$$t_{1/2} = t_{1/2N}/P \tag{5}$$

Based on these data individually adapted dosage regimens may be calculated according to one of the dosage rules published elsewhere [6].

It is intuitively clear that the decrease in drug elimination with decreasing renal function will be the more pronounced the larger the so-called standard renal dose fraction, f_{rN} (i. e. the fraction of the absorbed dose eliminated unchanged in the urine of the standard

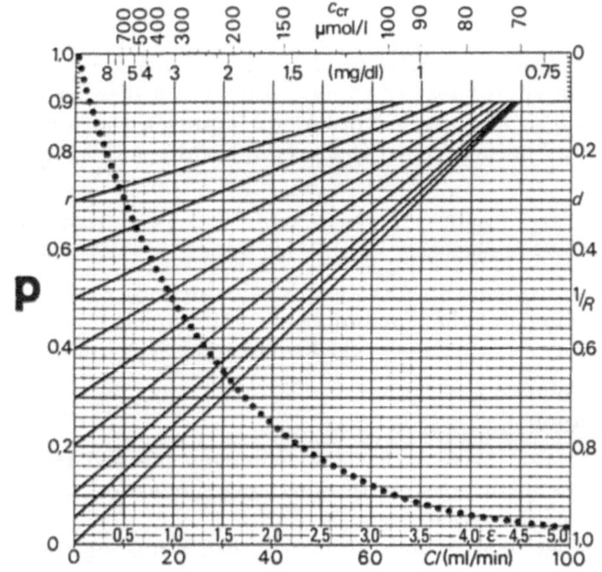

Fig. 1
Nomograph for the estimation of the individual clearance fraction of drugs, P_0, as a function of the endogenous creatinine clearance Cl. The use of the nomograph is explained in the text.

individual characterized by Cl = 100 ml/min) or the smaller the value of the minimal drug clearance fraction, $P_0 = \dot{V}_{nr}/\dot{V}_N$. Quantitative analysis of these relationships resulted in

$$P_0 = f_{nr} = 1 - f_{rN} \tag{6}$$

i. e. the minimal drug clearance fraction, P_0, which describes quantitatively the relationship between over-all drug clearance and creatinine clearance is numerically identical with the extra-renal dose fraction, f_{nr}. Since $f_{nr} = 1 - f_{rN}$ it follows that P_0 may de determined from the standard renal dose fraction, f_{rN}, by means of eq. 6. On the other hand we have demonstrated that the standard renal dose fraction, f_{rN}, may be calculated from the individual renal dose fraction, f_r, determined in any individual with or without renal impairment according to the following equation [4, 5]:

$$f_{rN} = \frac{Cl/Cl_N}{Cl/Cl_N + \dfrac{fr}{1 - fr}} \tag{7}$$

Eqs. 6 and 7 are of considerable practical importance because to determine the value P_0 of a drug from drug clearance measurements in the plasma elaborate and time-consuming kinetic experiments have to be performed in a large number of patients with renal disease of widely different degree. The possibility to determine P_0 in preclinical routine experiments from the renal dose fraction in individuals without renal disease contributed greatly to the fact that the values of P_0 of more than 600 drugs are presently known. These values are published in yearly intervals in an updated form in „Arzneimittelkompendium der Schweiz" [6].

Renal Function and Age

Kidney function as measured by the endogenous creatinine clearance, Cl, increases with age until a maximum is reached within approximately twenty years. From then on Cl decreases linearly by approximately 0.8 % per year. According to Biornsson the following equations describe the decrease in "normal" renal function in healthy adults with normal body weight [1]:

$$\text{Men:} \quad \text{Cl (ml/min)} = 143.5 - (1.095 \cdot \text{age}) \tag{8a}$$
$$\text{Women:} \quad \text{Cl (ml/min)} = 119.5 - (0.915 \cdot \text{age}) \tag{8b}$$

To give an impression of the quantitative consequences let us calculate two extreme values of "normal" renal function by means of the equations 8a and 8b, namely in a 20-year-old male and in a 90-year-old female of normal body weight. The result is as follows:

$$\text{20-year-old man:} \quad \text{Cl} = 122 \text{ ml/min}$$
$$\text{90-year-old women:} \quad \text{Cl} = 37 \text{ ml/min}$$

In view of this huge difference it appears evident that the frequently misused term "normal renal function" is meaning-less in the context of renal drug elimination when used without specifying at least the age of the patient.

The main reason that the influence of age is often underestimated when evaluating renal function in elderly patients is that the determination of Cl is usually impractical in the daily clinical setting. As a substitute it is customary to use the steady-state serum concentration of creatinine, c_{cr}, to characterize renal function. However, when c_{cr} is used as an estimate of the functional capacity of the kidneys the following kinetic facts should be considered: When a substance (e.g. a drug) is administered continuously at the infusion rate $\dot{D}$ its over-all clearance, $\dot{V}$, can be calculated from the steady-state plasma concentration, c_{ss}, eventually reached because c_{ss} is proportional to the infusion rate, $\dot{D}$, and inversely proportional to the drug clearance, $\dot{V}$:

$$c_{ss} = \dot{D}/\dot{V} \quad \text{or} \quad \dot{V} = \dot{D}/c_{ss} \tag{9}$$

Since reatinine is also produced at a constant rate, $\dot{m}$, creatinine clearance, Cl, can also be calculated in a similar way from $\dot{m}$ and the steady-state plasma creatinine concentration, c_{cr}, because

$$c_{cr} = \dot{m}/\text{Cl} \quad \text{or} \quad \text{Cl} = \dot{m}/c_{cr} \tag{10}$$

However, as a consequence of the decreasing muscular mass the creatinine production rate, $\dot{m}$, drcreases with age at about the same rate as does creatinine clearance, Cl. As predicted by eq. 10 c_{cr} will therefore remain practically constant throughout adult life in spite of the marked decrease in Cl. This means that plasma creatinine concentration per se is not a suitable parameter to adjust the dosage regimen of a drug to the functional capacity of the ageing kidney because c_{cr} may grossly over-estimate renal function. However, the problem can be solved reliably by using one of the well-known estimating equations that consider the influence of body weight, age, and sex on the relationship between c_{cr} and Cl. The best documented method is the estimating equation of Cockroft and Gault which reads as follows [3]:

$$\text{Cl} = \frac{(140 - \text{age}) \cdot \text{weight}}{72 \cdot c_{cr} \text{ (mg/dl)}} \tag{11}$$

The equation is valid for adult males; in females 15 % is subtracted from the result. Estimating Cl by means of eq. 11 proved to be even more reliable under clinical ward conditions than its direct measurement [8].

The following example reported by Follath [7] illustrates the situation: In 230 elderly patients without overt renal disease treated with 0.25 mg digoxin per day orally, objective signs of digoxin intoxication and toxic digoxin plasma concentrations where found in approximately 20 % of the patients. No relationship was found between the plasma creatinine concentration, c_{cr}, on the one hand and signs of toxicity or digoxin plasma concentration, c_{ss}, on the other. However, when Cl was estimated from c_{cr} according to eq. 11 all intoxicated patients had a creatinine clearance below 50 ml/min and an inverse hyperbolic relationship between digoxin plasma concentration, c_{ss}, and Cl was demonstrated as predicted by eq. 9. This is not an unexpected finding because the relatively low value $P_0 = 0.3$ for digoxin [6] indicates that the drug is eliminated predominantly (i. e. $f_{rN} = 0.7$) by the kidneys. As a consequence the over-all clearance of digoxin depends on renal function and will therefore be markedly smaller in the aged patient.

Finally, it should be emphasized that c_{cr} and eq. 11 should never be used to estimate Cl in patients with acute renal impairment or changing kidney function [4].

Extra-Renal Factors Influencing Renal Drug Elimination

The theory discussed in the present report does not consider extra-renal factors such as abnormal drug distribution which might influence renal drug elimination. In this respect the following age-related changes should be considered: During adult life an increase of body fat and a corresponding decrease of lean body mass takes place. Furthermore there is a decrease in total body water, extra-cellular water and plasma albumin concentration. As to be expected there is ample evidence in the literature that these age-related processes may markedly influence drug distribution. However, from a therapeutic point of view the clinical importance of these alterations in drug distribution should not be over-rated for the following reasons:

1. The main clinical concern is abnormal drug accumulation during repeated drug administration i. e. an abnormally high or abnormally low value of the mean steady-state plasma concentration, c_{ss}, due to an abnormal distribution volume, V. As can be seen from eq. 9 this is improbable because c_{ss} depends solely on the dose administered per time, $\dot{D}$, and on the over-all drug clearance, $\dot{V}$, and is independent of the distribution volume, V.

2. Regarding a drug bound to plasma albumin the pharmacological and toxicological activity depends on its unbound concentration. Since a lower than normal plasma albumin concentration means a lower than normal drug binding capacity and consequently a higher than normal unbound fraction, it is often concluded that the activity of a drug must be increased in states of hypoalbuminemia. In general this is not true, because when the unbound fraction increases, redistribution processes will result in a nearly normal unbound drug concentration and a lower than normal total drug plasma concentration.

3. The over-all elimination rate constant, k, and the biological half-life, $t_{1/2}$, of the drug depend in the following way on the distribution volume, V:

$$k = 0{,}693/t_{1/2} = \dot{V}/V \tag{12}$$

Since an increased unbound fraction of a drug results in a proportional increase of the distribution volume one would expect an increase in half-life. This if often not the case because many drug elimination mechanisms such as glomerular drug filtration are not proportional to total drug concentration but to unbound drug concentration. As a result the half-life remains unchanged. When a drug elimination process such as tubular secretion is proportional to total drug plasma concentration an increase in distribution volume will result in an increased half-life. However, it should be stated again that the steady-state drug plasma concentration, c_{ss}, eventually reached depends solely on drug clearance, $\dot{V}$, and is independent of the distribution volume, V, as predicted by eq. 9.

It follows from these considerations that, from a clinical point of view, age-related abnormal drug distribution is usually of minor importance although it may markedly influence some characteristics (e. g. the half-life) of the drug plasma concentration curve. For drugs eliminated pre-dominantly by the kidneys the age related decrease in renal clearance is therefore by far the most important kinetic abnormality in the elderly patient.

Conclusion

In adult patients without renal disease the renal clearance and consequently the over-all clearance of drugs eliminated predominantly by the kidneys decreases markedly with age. As drug clearance is the most important determinant of drug accumulation the mean steady-state drug plasma concentration in the elderly may be considerably higher than in young patients when the dosage regimen is not modified accordingly. It appears that the therapeutic index of most commonly used drugs is so large, that overt signs of toxicity are not seen in the majority of old patients. Nevertheless it is reasonable to assume that an abnormally high steady-state drug plasma concentration increases the risk of side effects and undoubtedly contributes to the generally accepted fact that adverse drug reactions are considerably more common in the elderly. At least in the following critical situations the functional capacity of the kidneys should be estimated and the dosage regimen should be quantitatively modified according to the simple methods described in this report:

1. When the drug has a low value of P_0 and at the same time a small therapeutic index. Examples are digoxin ($P_0 = 0.3$) and the aminoglycosides ($P_0 < 0.02$).
2. In the presence of concomitant pathology such as dehydration, cachexia, low fluid intake etc., which is much more common in old than in young patients.

References

[1] *Biornsson, T. D.*: Clin. Pharmacokin. 4, 200, 1979.
[2] *Bricker, N. S.*: Amer. J. Med. 28, 77, 1960.
[3] *Cockroft, D. W., Gault, H.*: Nephron 16, 31, 1976.
[4] *Dettli, L.*: Elimination Kinetics and Dosage Adjustment of Drugs in Patients with Kidney Disease. Fischer, New York 1977.
[5] *Dettli, L.*: Jap. J. clin. Pharmacol. Ther. 15, 241, 1984.
[6] *Dettli, L., Galeazzi, R. L.*: Pharmakokinetische Grundlagen der Arzneimitteldosierung, in Arzneimittelkompendium der Schweiz. Documed, Basel 1985.
[7] *Follath, F.*: Fortschr. Med. 100, 1431, 1982.
[8] *Wheeler, L. A., Sheiner, L. B.*: Amer. J. clin. Pathol. 72, 27, 1979.

III Specific Drug Treatment

Anti-anginal Therapy in the Aged

W. Schneider

Zentrum der Inneren Medizin, Abteilung für Kardiologie, Klinikum der Johann
Wolfgang Goethe-Universität, Theodor Stern-Kai 7, D-6000 Frankfurt am Main

Summary

The generally accepted principles of anti-anginal therapy can also be applied to the
elderly. The circulatory system of the geriatric patient however shows decreased
adaptation to exogenous influences including drugs with vasodilating or negative
inotropic properties. Thus gradual dosage adaptation is mandatory and withdrawal
or dose reduction should be considered if adverse effects occur.
The pharmacokinetic parameters of commonly used anti-anginal drugs allow for
normal dosages in most elderly subjects. Problems may be caused by hydrophilic
β-blockers in the elderly with impaired renal function. Dose reduction is sometimes
advisable with calcium antagonists.
Of the variety of currently available anti-anginal drugs, nitrates are of outstanding
value for acute and chronic treatment. Calcium channel blockers are gaining importance and are especially beneficial if hypertensive patients are to be treated.
β-blockers should be used with caution in the elderly. Patients with severe angina
should receive double- or triple combination therapy.

Introduction

General principles of antianginal therapy with organic nitrates, calcium channel blocking
agents and beta-sympatholytic drugs are valid in the management of the geriatric patient.
However, decrease in the adaptation of the cardiovascular system in the elderly should
be taken into account. Of the large variety of physiological features in advanced age, loss
of elasticity of blood vessels, increased (systolic) blood pressure, decrease of intrinsic
heart rate and reduced adaptation of hemodynamics to physical stress should be mentioned
[15, 16, 25]. Thus the probability of adverse drug effects is increased.
As far as electrophysiological functions are concerned it should be noted that the atrio-
ventricular conduction time, represented by the PQ-interval in the ECG, increases by
10 ms every decade after the age of 20 [25].
Some basic considerations are noteworthy with regard to absorption, distribution,
metabolism and elimination of antianginal drugs: Drug absorption in the GI tract is
generally a passive process (diffusion) and no impairment is expected in the elderly [21].
The increase of fat tissue and the corresponding decrease of the extracellular volume,
plasma water and total body water in old age explains the increased volume of distribution (V_D) for lipophilic agents (e.g. propranolol) and the decreased volume of distribution for highly water-soluble compounds (e.g. atenolol) [20, 21]. Decreased kidney
clearance in the geriatric patient may occasionally cause problems after sustained use of
hydrophylic agents (e.g. atenolol) [2, 5, 8, 20, 21, 33].

So far there are no data available suggesting the need for dosage adjustment in the elderly with impaired hepatic function and decreased plasma protein binding [4, 21, 26, 31].
From a practical point of view it is important to recognize that the clinical symptoms in old patients with cardiovascular diseases may be atypical where dyspnoea, dizziness, indigestion and gastrointestinal complaints are the leading symptoms [16, 23, 25].

Organic Nitrates

The organic nitrates are the first-line drugs for the treatment of angina pectoris in the elderly. They act primarily by increasing blood pooling in the venous capacitance vessels and enhancing elasticity of the large elastic-type arteries. Thus cardiac pre- and afterload are reduced with a concomitant decrease of ventricular filling pressures, wall tension and oxygen consumption [28].
After oral dosage isosorbide dinitrate (ISDN) and glyceryl trinitrate (GTN) undergo hepatic first-pass metabolism with splitting off of nitrate groups [6,9,11,29]. Bioavailability of ISDN after intestinal absorption is as low as 20 % [6]. The hydrophilic pharmacologically active main metabolite of ISDN isosorbide-5-mononitrate (IS-5-MN), is subject to a very weak hepatic degradation and thus exhibits a long elimination half-life (plasma $t_{1/2}$ = 4.5 hours) [4, 6, 9]. Prior to renal elimination the metabolites of ISDN (isosorbide, isosorbide-2- and isosorbide-5-mononitrate) are bound to glucuronic acid [4, 6, 9]. Commonly used nitrates such as GTN, ISDN and IS-5-MN are characterized by a large volume of distribution (V_D): 0.34 l/kg (GTN), 0.65 l/kg (IS-5-MN) and 1.8 l/kg (ISDN) [22]. Obviously nitrates are considerably accumulated in vessel walls [14].
Despite a predominantly renal elimination no cumulation phenomena have been seen so far for ISDN and the mononitrate metabolites [4]. In patients with hepatic failure of various degrees neither cumulation nor metabolism abnormalities could be detected for ISDN or its metabolites [39].
Due to the smaller volume of distribution of the relatively hydrophilic isosorbide-5-mononitrate its plasma-concentrations may be somewhat elevated in the elderly.
Our own data in 14 patients being treated with ISDN 40 mg q.i.d. for 2 weeks revealed only a 15 % difference in mean plasma concentrations between the younger (51—59 years) and older (60—71 years) subgroup (Fig. 1) [34].
Thus dosage adjustment of ISDN and isosorbide-5-mononitrate in the aged even with impaired renal and hepatic function is rarely necessary. A further important aspect of nitrate therapy in the elderly is the responsiveness of arterial blood pressure and heart rate after acute administration. In patients not accustomed to nitrates a marked drop of arterial blood pressure in the upright position is expected. However there are no data providing evidence for a more pronounced hypotensive reaction in the elderly: Westermann and co-workers (1976) described a 17—18 % decrease of systolic blood pressure after 20 mg ISDN administered sublingually regardless of the age [42]. Nevertheless one should be aware of a reduced tolerance to hypotension in the geriatric patient with impaired autoregulation of cerebral blood flow [25]. During sustained nitrate therapy the circulatory effects are mild and rarely cause problems even in hypotensive patients.

Application form and doses (Fig. 2):

1. The acute anginal attack is best treated with sublingual nitroglycerin. In the aged 0.4 mg often provide prompt relief without hazardous circulatory effects. Dose

augmentation is advisable in severe attacks. Nitroglycerin sprays will give similar results. Long-lasting attacks and unstable angina are best treated by nitroglycerin via the intravenous route. Hourly doses of 1.5–3.0 (− 6.0) mg are recommended. Continous circulatory monitoring is mandatory.

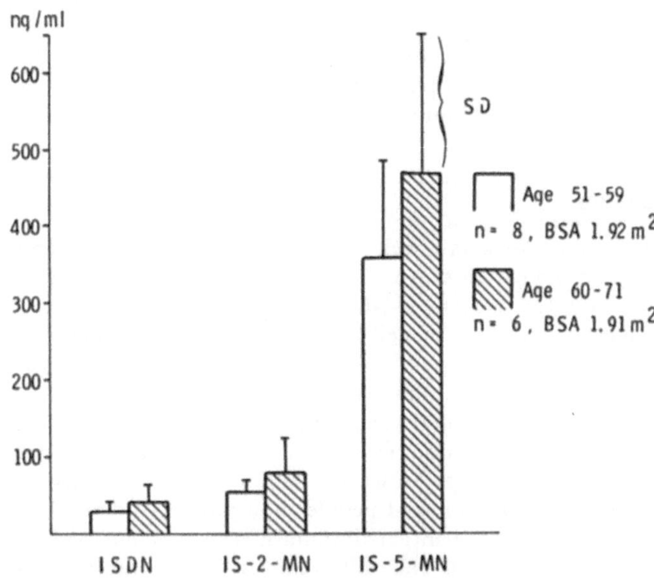

Fig. 1
Age-related mean plasma concentrations of isosorbide dinitrate (ISDN) and the mononitrate metabolites after 2-week treatment with ISDN 40 mg t.i.d. Determination of plasma concentrations 60 min after first dose on day 14. (Mean values + SD)

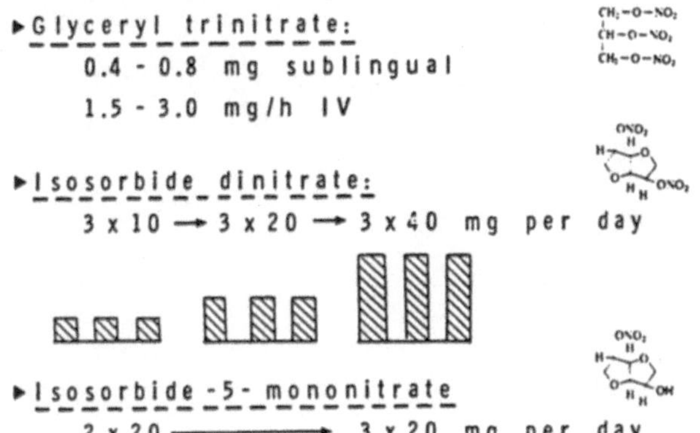

Fig. 2
Recommended doses of glyceryl trinitrate (GTN), isosorbide dinitrate (ISDN) and isosorbide-5-mononitrate in the elderly. Gradual dose augmentation is advisable corresponding to the severity of angina.

2. Most old patients with stable angina due to fixed and dynamic coronary obstructions
   benefit from long-term therapy with isosorbide dinitrate and isosorbide-5-mono-
   nitrate. Initially single doses of 10 mg isosorbide dinitrate t.i.d. or 20 mg isosorbide-5-
   mononitrate b.i.d. are recommended. Mean standard doses in long-term therapy are
   3 X 20 mg isosorbide dinitrate or 2—3 X 20 mg isosorbide-5-mononitrate. In severe
   angina dosage increase is useful: 3 X 40 mg isosorbide dinitrate per day.

Single doses of 20—40 mg isosorbide dinitrate or 20 mg isosorbide-5-mononitrate in
standard formulation administered 2—4 times a day are supposed to maintain their efficacy during long-term therapy [34, 35]. Nitroglycerin patches applied once daily for 12
hours may be therapeutically effective in old people with mild angina too. Their therapeutic value in long-term therapy is not yet determined.

Calcium channel-blocking agents

The antianginal value of calcium channel blockers is well recognised in antianginal therapy
irrespective of the type of angina and the patients' age. They act by decreasing peripheral
vascular resistance (→ reduction of afterload), by dilating dynamic coronary stenoses
and spasms and by direct influencing the myocardial cell (e.g. preservation of high-energy
triphosphates).
A mild negative inotropic effect is of minor clinical importance [23].
In the old patient the maintained sympatho-neural circulatory control during calcium
channel blocker therapy is advantageous. In addition, most coronary patients will benefit
from the pressure-lowering effects of these drugs. However, the increased sensitivity of
blood pressure response to calcium antagonists in old people should be considered [7].
A number of patients obtain advantage from the anti-arrhythmic effects of some calcium
channel-blockers, such as verapamil, gallopamil and diltiazem. Recently interest has
focussed on the potentially beneficial effects of these drugs on the formation and
progression of atheroscloretic lesions [17] (Tab. I).
The pharmacokinetic profile of the commonly used calcium antagonists deserves some
comment:
Nifedipine, a dihydropyridine compound, is characterized by a bioavailability of about
65 % after intestinal absorption [18]. Approximately 90 % of the drug is protein-bound
[18]. Elimination half-life is reported to be 4—5 hours after oral administration [18].
Pharmacological effects depend on plasma concentrations higher than 40 ng/ml [3]. So

Table I: Advantages of antianginal therapy with calcium antagonists in geriatrix patients.

A D V A N T A G E S   I N   O L D   A G E

▶ Prevention of coronary spasms

▶ Preservation of adrenergic regulation

▶ Antiarrhythmic effects

▶ Reduction of arterial blood pressure

▶ Slowing of atherosclerosis ?

far no evidence for drug accumulation during sustained therapy has been provided [3].

The molecular structure of verapamil shows some similarities to papaverine. The drug undergoes extensive hepatic first-pass metabolism after oral administration. Thus the bioavailability is only 20 % [19].

The pharmacological activity of the metabolite norverapamil is about 20 % as compared with the parent compound [30]. Plasma protein-binding is high: 90 % [43]. Elimination half-life is 4 hours after a single dose and 10—12 hours after chronic administration [27, 37]. Prolonged elimination half-life and increased bioavailability are found in patients with impaired hepatic function [38, 43].

The drug is well-tolerated: the range of therapeutic plasma concentrations starts with 40 ng/ml (effects on AV-conduction) and extends to 200 ng/ml [13]. Plasma concentrations exceeding 900 ng/ml have been reported without adverse effects [13].

Abernethy and co-workers reported a 60 % reduction of verapamil clearance with age [1]. Own data from 14 patients treated for 2 weeks with 120 mg verapamil t.i.d. revealed no differences in mean plasma concentrations between the younger (51—59 years) and older (60—71 years) subgroup (Fig. 3) [34].

Thus administration of mean maintenance doses of this calcium channel blocker will not generally be accompanied by accumulation and dose adjustment in the elderly is rarely necessary [40].

The structure of diltiazem is related to the benzodiazepines. The drug is well-absorbed (95 %) via the intestinal mucosa [24, 26]. 80 % of the compound is protein-bound [26]. Liver metabolism plays an important role in drug elimination [26] and an entero-hepatic circulation has been described [32]. From previous studies it is known that elimination half-life is somewhat prolonged in the elderly [26].

Since AV-conduction time gradually increases with age, drugs with negative dromotropic effects like verapamil, gallopamil and diltiazem should be used with caution in geriatric patients. Individuals with sinus node and AV-node disorders should be excluded from

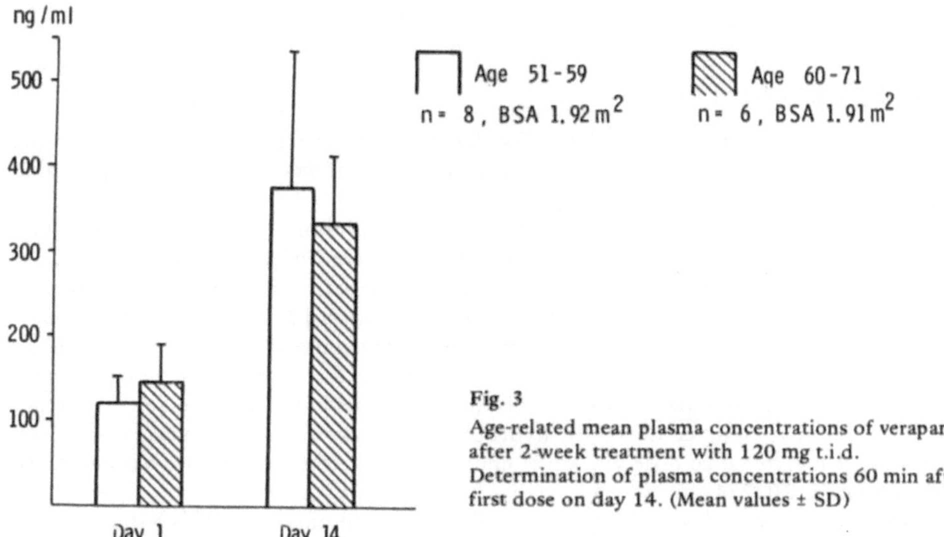

Fig. 3
Age-related mean plasma concentrations of verapamil after 2-week treatment with 120 mg t.i.d.
Determination of plasma concentrations 60 min after first dose on day 14. (Mean values ± SD)

Table II: Recommended daily doses of the most commonly used calcium antagonists in the elderly. Gallopamil is a methoxy derivative of verapamil.

CALCIUM ANTAGONISTS

Recommended doses in the elderly

1. VERAPAMIL
3 x 80 mg
3 x 120 mg

Verapamil (Isoptin)

2. GALLOPAMIL
3 x 25 mg
3 x 50 mg

Gallopamil (Procorum)

3. NIFEDIPINE
3 x 10 mg
3 x 20 mg s. r.

Nifedipin (Adalat)

4. DILTIAZEM
3 x 60 mg

Diltiazem (Dilzem)

therapy and be treated with drugs without such profile (e. g. nifedipine).

Nevertheless therapy with the aforementioned drugs with negative dromotropic effects is associated with a low risk in the elderly if ECG monitoring is routinely performed 60—90 minutes after an initial high oral dose.

For the commonly used calcium antagonistic drugs, the following daily doses are recommended (Table II).

β-adrenergic Blocking Agents

β-blockers exert their anti-anginal effects by decreasing heart rate (negative chronotropic effect) and by reducing wall stress (negative inotropic effect). As a result myocardial performance and oxygen demand are diminished [2, 8].

At present a large variety of β-blockers are available for clinical use. The pharmacokinetic parameters of the different compounds show considerable differences (Table III): lipophilic agents such as propranolol undergo extensive hepatic first-pass metabolism and elimination is relatively independent from kidney function [2, 5, 12, 20]. In contrast, hydrophilic agents such as atenolol are predominantly eliminated by the kidney [20]. Thus drugs with long plasma half-lives and mainly renal excretion may accumulate during long-term therapy in old patients especially in individuals with impaired renal function [20, 21]. In clinical practice dosage of hydrophilic β-blockers should be reduced by 50 % of a standard maintenance dose whenever endogenous creatinine clearance has decreased to 30 ml/min [5, 20, 21].

Some authors have stated that the number of β-receptors in human heart is reduced in old age [36] and that the susceptibility towards β-blocking agents might be weaker [41]. So

Table III: Some pharmacokinetic features of β-blocking drugs: propranolol is mainly metabolised in the liver. Its hydrophilic degradation products, with only residual pharmacological activity, undergo renal elimination. Kidney function is of major importance in hydrophilic compounds (atenolol, nadolol, sotalol).

ß - B L O C K E R S   I N   O L D   A G E

PHARMACOKINETICS

● First - Pass - Effect / Lipophilia
   Propranolol

● Protein binding
   Propranolol : 85 - 95 %
   Metoprolol : 10 %

● Renal excretion
   hydrophilic agents
   Atenolol : 100 %
   Nadolol : 100 %
   Sotalol : 60 - 90 %

   Propranolol ⟶ hydrophilic metabolites

Table IV: Advantages and disadvantages of β-blockers in old age.

ß - B L O C K E R S   I N   O L D   A G E

ADVANTAGES

▶ Lowering of blood pressure

▶ Possible antiarrhythmic effects

PROBLEMS

▶ Bradykardia

▶ Bronchial resistance ↑

▶ Heart failure

▶ Filling pressures
  Peripheral resistance ↑

▶ Metabolic side effects

far these observations have not influenced practical application of these drugs in the aged. β-blockers like Calcium antagonists favourably influence blood pressure in the hypertensive patient with coronary artery disease [10]. The non-specific membrane stabilizing effect may be desirable in patients with rhythm disturbances. On the other hand the drugs may be hazardous in patients with bradycardia, bronchial, asthma, impaired left venticular function and peripheral vascular disease. Such patients should be excluded from β-blocker therapy. The contraindications refer to non-selective and β_1-selective compounds [2, 5, 12, 21] (Table IV).

Therapy schedule in the elderly (Table V)

Nitrates are the first-choice drugs for the treatment of angina pectoris in the elderly. Their clinical value is high in the treatment of acute anginal attacks and in long-term therapy.
Clincal interest in calcium channel blockers is increasing due to their additional antihypertensive effects and their protective role in myocardial cell metabolism. β-blockers should be used with care in the elderly.
Combination therapy is often mandatory in the geriatric patient: Nitrates can be favourably combined with calcium channel-blocking agents and β-blockers. The combination of nitrates with nifedipine and other calcium antagonists without negative dromotropic effects may cause tachycardia via reflex mechanisms. Thus nitrates should preferrably be combined with verapamil, gallopamil or diltiazem.
In patients with severe angina pectoris triple-combination (nitrates, calcium channel blockers, β-blockers) is recommended. β-blockers should not be combined with verapamil, gallopamil (or diltiazem) in the elderly due to potential conduction disturbances.

Table V: Therapy schedule for the treatment of angina pectoris in the elderly.

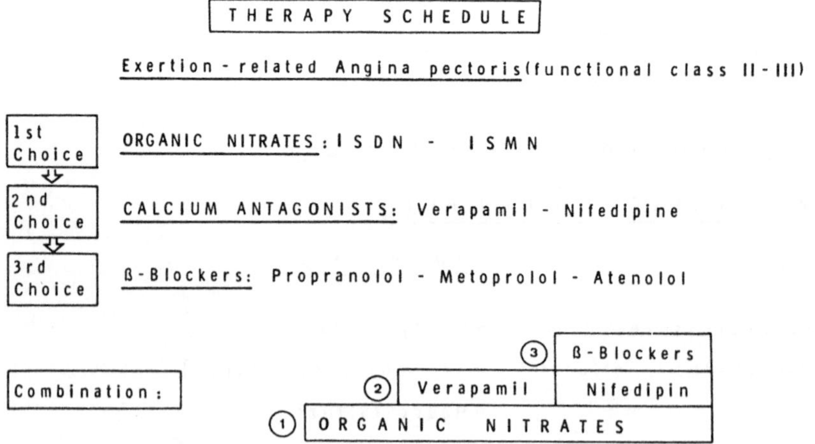

Specific Therapeutic Considerations (Table VI)

Nitrates can be safely combined with nifedipine for the management of old people with angina pectoris and bradycardia. On the other hand verapamil and β-blockers have value in patients with tachycardia. Hypertensive patients should always receive combination therapy, preferrably with nitrates and calcium channel blocking agents.
The geriatric patient with hypotension should be treated with care: Incremental doses of nitrates often allow gradual adaptation of circulatory regulation.
Nitrates and calcium blockers are the drugs of choice in patients with vasospastic angina. β-blockers may be detrimental in these individuals.

Table VI: Specific therapeutic considerations in the elderly with angina pectoris and associated problems.

SPECIFIC THERAPEUTIC CONSIDERATIONS

ANGINA PECTORIS

+ Bradykardia	⟶	Nitrates / Nifedipine
+ Tachykardia	⟶	Verapamil / ß - Blockers / (Nitrates)
+ Hypertension	⟶	Nitrates / Calcium antag. / ß-Blockers
+ Hypotension	⟶	Nitrates (incremental doses)
+ Vasospasm	⟶	Nitrates / Calcium antagonists
+ Heart failure	⟶	Nitrates / Calcium antagonists Diuretics / Digitalis

Nitrates and calcium antagonists may be used without problems in patients with angina pectoris and heart failure. β-blockers should be avoided. Additional therapy with diuretic drugs, digitalis and if necessary ACE-inhibitors or other vasodilating drugs is recommended.

References

[1] *Abernethy, D. R., Schwartz, J. B., Todd, E. L., Luchi, R., Snow, E.:* Pharmacodynamics and disposition of racemic verapamil in elderly and very elderly hypertensive patients. Clin. Pharmacol. Ther. **37**, 177 astr. (1985).

[2] *Ablad, B.:* β-blockers: theory, action, and application to the elderly. In: Beta-blockers in the elderly. Lang, E., Sörgel, F., Blaha, L. (eds.) Springer-Verlag, Berlin, Heidelberg, New York, p. 3–22 (1982).

. [3] *Aoki, K., Sato, K., Kawaguchi, Y., Yamamoto, M.:* Acute and long-term hypotensive effects and plasma concentrations of nifedipine in patients with essential hypertension. Eur. J. Clin. Pharmacol. **23**, 197–201, (1982).

[4] *Bogaert, M. G., Rosseel, M. T., Boelaert, J., Daneels, R.:* Fate of isosorbide dinitrate and mononitrates in patients with renal failure. Eur. J. Clin. Pharmacol. **21**, 73–76, (1981).

[5] *Bolte, H. D.:* Betarezeptorenblocker. Pharmakokinetik und therapeutische Wirksamkeit. Internist. **23**, 616–623, (1982).

[6] *Bonn, R.:* Pharmakokinetik organischer Nitrate unter besonderer Berücksichtigung von Isosorbid-5-nitrat. In: Mononitrat. 2. Workshop Kronberg, 1983. Köhler, E., Noack, E., Schrey, A., Weiß, M. (eds.). Universitätsdruckerei und Verlag Dr. C. Wolf und Sohn, München p. 24–37, (1983).

[7] *Bühler, F., Hulthén, U. L., Kiowski, W., Müller, F. B., Bolli, P.:* The place of the calcium antagonist verapamil in antihypertensive therapy. J. cardiovasc. Pharmacol. **4**, Suppl. **3**, 350–357, (1982).

[8] *Castleden, C. M., George, C. F.:* The effect of ageing on the hepatic clearance of propranolol. Br. J. Clin. Pharmacol. **7**, 49–54, (1979).

[9] *Chasseaud, L. F., Wood, S. G., Luckow, V.:* Metabolism von ^{14}C-Isosorbid-5-mononitrat. In: Mononitrat. 2. Workshop Kronberg 1983. Köhler, E., Noack, E., Schrey, A., Weiß, M. (eds.). Universitätsdruckerei und Verlag Dr. C. Wolf und Sohn München, p. 49–59, (1983).

[10] *Conway, J., Wheeler, R., Sannerstedt, R.:* Sympathetic nervous activity during exercise in relation to age. Cardiovasc. Res. **5**, 577, (1971).

[11] *Down, W. H., Chasseaud, L. F., Grundy, R. K.:* Biotransformation of isosorbide dinitrate in humans. J. Pharm. Sci. **63**, 1147–1149, (1974).

[12] *Estler, C. J., Sörgel, F.:* Pharmacokinetics of β-blockers in the elderly. In: Beta-blockers in the elderly. Lang, E., Sörgel, F., Blaha, L. (eds.). Springer-Verlag Berlin, Heidelberg, New York, p. 23–32, (1982).

[13] *Frishman, W., Kirsten, E., Klein, M., Pine, M., Johnson, S. M., Hillis, L. D., Packer, M., Kates, R.:* Clinical relevance of verapamil plasma levels in stable angina pectoris. Am. J. Cardiol. **50**, 1180–1184, (1982).

[14] *Fung, H. L., Sutton, S. C., Kamiya, A.:* Blood vessel uptake and metabolism of organic nitrates in the rat. J. Pharmacol, exp. Therap. **228**, 334–341, (1984).

[15] *Gerstenblith, G., Lakatta, E. G., Weisfeld, M. D.:* Age changes in myocardial function and exercise response. Prog. Cardiovasc. Dis. **19**, 1–21, (1976).

[16] *Harris, R.:* Cardiovascular diseases in the elderly. Med. Clin. N. Amer. **67**, 379–394, (1983).

[17] *Henry, P. D.:* Atherosclerosis, calcium, and calcium antagonists. Circulation **72**, 456–459, (1985).

[18] *Horster, F. A.:* Pharmacokinetics of nifedipine-^{14}C in man. In: The second international Adalat Symposium. Lochner, W., Braasch, W., Kroneberg, G. (eds.). Springer-Verlag, New York, 49–54, (1975).

[19] *Johnston, A., Burgess, C. D., Hamer, J.:* Systemic availability of oral verapamil and effect on PR interval in man. Br. J. Clin. Pharmacol. **12**, 397–400, (1981).

[20] *Kirch, W., Köhler, H., Mutschler, E., Schäfer, M.:* Pharmacokinetics of atenolol in relation to renal function. Europ. J. Clin. Pharmacol. **19**, 65–71, (1981).

[21] *Klaus, W.:* Pharmakologisch-therapeutische Besonderheiten im Alter, speziell auf dem Gebiet der Herz-Kreislaufkrankheiten. Z. Kardiol. 75, Suppl. **7**, 27–31, (1985).

[22] *Klotz, U.:* Klinische Pharmakokinetik. Gustav Fischer Verlag, Stuttgart, New York, 2. Auflage, 1984.

[23] *Kober, G.:* Koronare Herzkrankheit: Wie zeigt sie sich im Alter? Ärztl. Prax. **23**, 3665–3667, (1981).

[24] *Kohno, K., Takenchi, Y., Etoh, A., Noda, K.:* Pharmacokinetics and bioavailability of diltiazem (CRD-401) in dog. Arzneim. Forsch. (Drug. Res.) **27**, 1424–1428, (1977).

[25] *Lang, E.:* Klinisch-pharmakologische und therapeutische Besonderheiten der geriatrischen Kardiologie. Z. Altersforsch. **38**, 369–375, (1983).

[26] *Morselli, P. L., Rovei, V., Mitchard, M., Durand, A., Gomeni, R., Larriband, J.:* Pharmacokinetics and metabolism of diltiazem in man (observations on healthy volunteers and angina pectoris patients). In: New drug therapy with a calcium antagonist: Diltiazem Hakone Symposium. 1978. Bing, R. J. (ed.). Excerpta Medica, Amsterdam, p. 152–167, 1978.

[27] *McAllister, R. G., Jr.:* Clinical pharmacology of slow channel blocking agents. Prog. Cardiovasc. Dis. **25**, 83–102, (1982).

[28] *McGregor, M.:* The nitrates and myocardial ischemia. Circulation. **66**, 689–692, (1982).

[29] *Needleman, P., Harkey, A. M.:* Role of endogenous glutathione in the metabolism of glyceryl trinitrate by isolated perfused rat liver. Biochem. Pharmacol. **20**, 1867–1976, (1971).

[30] *Neugebauer, G.:* Comparative cardiovascular actions of verapamil and its major metabolites in the anesthetized dog. Cardiovasc. Res. **12**, 247–254, (1978).

[31] *Ochs, H. R., Verburg-Ochs, B.:* Einfluß von Alter, Gewicht, Geschlecht und Rauchgewohnheiten auf die Medikamentendosierung. Internist. **24**, 167–181, (1983).

[32] *Piepho, R. W., Bloedow, D. C., Lacz, J. P., Runser, D. J., Dimmit, D. C., Browne, R. K.:* Pharmacokinetics of diltiazem in selected animal species and human beings. Am. J. Cardiol. **49**, 525–528, (1982).

[33] *Platt, D.:* Drug treatment in the aged. In: Platt, D. (ed.). Geriatrics 2, Springer-Verlag, Berlin, p. 448–465, 1983.

[34] *Schneider, W., Lang, E., Woodcock, B., Kaltenbach, M.:* Acute and long-term effects of verapamil and isosorbide dinitrate (ISDN) in patients with angina pectoris. Eur. Heart J. (in press).

[35] *Schneider, W., Wietschoreck, A., Bußmann, W. D., Kaltenbach, M.:* Die anti-anginöse Wirksamkeit von Isosorbiddinitrat im akuten Versuch und nach einer 4-wöchigen Dauertherapie mit 6 × 40 mg pro Tag. Klin. Wochenschr. **63**, 460–467, (1985).

[36] *Schocken, D. D., Roth, G. S.:* Reduced β-adrenergic receptor concentration in ageing man. Nature **267**, 856–858, (1977).

[37] *Schwartz, J. B., Keefe, D. L., Kirsten, E., Kates, R. E., Harrison, D. C.:* Prolongation of verapamil elimination kinetics during chronic oral administration. Am. Heart J. **104**, 198–203, (1982).

[38] *Somogyi, A., Albrecht, M., Kliems, G., Schafer, K., Eichelbaum, M.:* Pharmacokinetics, bio-availability and ECG response of verapamil in patients with liver cirrhosis. Br. J. Clin. Pharmacol. **12**, 51—60, (1981).

[39] *Steudel, H., Volkenandt, M., Steudel, A. Th.:* Pharmacokinetics of isosorbide-5-mononitrate after oral and intravenous administration in patients with liver cirrhosis: first results. Z. Kardiol. 72, Suppl. **3**, 24—28, (1983).

[40] *Storstein, L., Larsen, A., Midtbø, K., Soevareid, L.:* Pharmacokinetics of calcium blockers in patients with renal insufficiency and in geriatric patients. Acta. Medica. Scand. Suppl. **681**, 25—30, (1983).

[41] *Vestal, R. E., Wood, A. J. J., Shand, D. G.:* Reduced β-adrenergic sensitivity in the elderly. Clin. Pharm. Ther. **26**, 181—186, (1979).

[42] *Westermann, K. W., Bischoff, K., Kugler, G., Schnabel, A.:* Die Wirkung von Isosorbiddinitrat in Abhängigkeit von Körperlage und Lebensalter. Z. Kardiol. **65** (976), 1060—1070.

[43] *Woodcock, B. G., Rietbrock, I., Vohringer, H. F., Rietbrock, N.:* Verapamil disposition in liver disease and intensive-care patients: Kinetics, clearance and apparent blood flow relationships. Clin. Pharmacol. Ther. **29**, 27—34, (1981).

Besonderheiten der Theophyllinkinetik im Alter: Welche Konsequenzen ergeben sich bei der Therapie obstruktiver Atemwegserkrankungen?

A. H. Staib

Abteilung für Klinische Pharmakologie, Klinikum der Johann Wolfgang Goethe-Universität Frankfurt, Theodor-Stern-Kai 7, D-6000 Frankfurt am Main 70

Zusammenfassung

1. Die Behandlung des Asthma bronchiale und anderer obstruktiver Atemwegserkrankungen weist bei älteren Patienten Besonderheiten auf. Der Einsatz von Theophyllinpräparaten muß hierbei weniger aus substanzspezifischen Veränderungen der Kinetik (geringere Proteinbindung, Verkleinerung des Verteilungsvolumens) als aus im Alter häufigeren indirekt wirksamen Faktoren unter kontrollierten Bedingungen erfolgen.
2. Die alterstypischen Faktoren, die eine Dosisindividualisierung erfordern, sind Parallelerkrankungen, häufigere Mehrfachmedikation, unbekanntes Ausmaß der Vormedikation. Diese führen in der Regel zu einer Verminderung der Theophyllin-Metabolisierung und erfordern deshalb eine Dosisreduktion.
3. Das Ausmaß der Dosisreduktion kann für ein einzelnen Patienten analog den Verhältnissen bei jüngeren Schwerkranken nicht vorausgesagt werden.
4. Diese grundsätzliche Dosierungsunsicherheit erfordert beim alten Menschen eine an Wirkung und Serumkonzentration orientierte Therapieüberwachung.

Summary

1. There exist age-dependent problems in the theophylline treatment of bronchial asthma and other chronic obstructive lung diseases.
2. Polymorbidity, multimedication, unknown premedication and rapid changes in the clinical stage of aged patients are important, but not substance specific kinetic changes such as decrease of V_d.
3. The dose changes needed are not predictable.
4. Therapeutic drug monitoring in the elderly is necessary for dosage optimisation.

Erkrankungen des Respirationstraktes gehören zu den wichtigsten zu Arbeitsausfall und Frühberentung führenden Krankheitsursachen. Die Therapie dieser Erkrankungen beansprucht deshalb besonderes Interesse.

Der therapeutische Einsatz von Theophyllin bei Störungen der Atmungsfunktion beruht in allen Altersgruppen auf den gleichen Grundwirkungen. Die Behandlung von obstruktiven Respirationsstörungen ist das dominierende Indikationsgebiet (Ausnahme: Apnoe-Syndrom des Früh- und Mangelgeborenen). Für die Akutbehandlung des Asthma bronchiale und der obstruktiven Bronchitis stellen Methylxanthine, besonders Theophyllin, seit Jahrzehnten [1, 2] ein bewährtes und besonders im Notfall praktisch unumstrittenes

Therapieprinzip dar. Für die Dauertherapie und die Prophylaxe sind Theophyllinpräparate nach oder neben β_2-Mimetika und vor Anticholinergika und Antiallergika Mittel der Wahl. Der Einsatz erfolgt entweder als Infusion oder oral (Lösung) bei akuter Verschlechterung der respiratorischen Funktion oder als orale Dauermedikation (Retardpräparate) zur Obstruktionsprophylaxe.

Hauptproblem einer rationalen Theophyllinanwendung ist die Notwendigkeit einer individuellen Dosierung, da nur so eine optimale Wirkung bei genügender therapeutischer Sicherheit garantiert werden kann. Dazu ist eine an klinischer Wirkung und Theophyllin-Serumkonzentration orientierte Dosisanpassung erforderlich.

Grundlage dieser heute klinisch allgemein akzeptierten Forderung ist die geringe therapeutische Breite (ausgedrückt als Verhältnis der Plasmakonzentrationsschwelle für antiobstruktive Wirkungen und der Konzentration, bei der eine nicht mehr vertretbare Inzidenz von unerwünschten Wirkungen vorhanden ist) und die nicht vorhersagbare inter- und intraindividuelle Variabilität der Eliminationsgeschwindigkeit für Theophyllin.

Für die therapeutische Anwendung ergeben sich beim älteren Menschen außer diesen für alle Altersstufen gültigen Faktoren weitere Aspekte für die Therapieführung:

1. zusätzlich zu exogenen Ursachen einer respiratorischen Störung (Allergie, Infektion ect.) treten mit zunehmender Krankheitsdauer und zunehmendem Alter irreversible morphologische Veränderungen auf (Emphysem), die das Substrat für den erwünschten pharmakodynamischen Effekt (Broncholyse) reduzieren können.

2. Die Multimorbidität des älteren Patienten erfordert häufig den Einsatz unterschiedlicher Pharmaka. Dadurch ist die Möglichkeit von Interaktionen, unerwünschten Wirkungen, Compliance-Schwierigkeiten etc. erhöht.

3. Elimination und andere kinetische Parameter des Theophyllins können sich als Erkrankungsfolge, durch Interaktionen mit anderen Arzneimitteln oder aus nicht abklärbaren Gründen rasch und nicht vorhersehbar ändern.

4. Soziale Faktoren sowie altersbedingte psychische und intellektuelle Veränderungen beeinträchtigen zunehmend Übersicht und Zuverlässigkeit des Patienten hinsichtlich einer erforderlichen Arzneimittelanwendung. Bei Substanzen mit kritischer therapeutischer Breite und/oder vitaler Indikation sind hierbei Probleme zu erwarten.

Die klinische Situation charakterisiert folgender Fall (Abb. 1):

Ein 78jähriger Patient wird wegen akuter respiratorischer und kardialer Insuffizienz auf die interne Intensivstation der Universitätsklinik aufgenommen. Bei unbekannter Theophyllinanamnese Routineinfusion eines Theophyllinpräparates (Euphyllin®) wegen schwerer obstruktiver Respirationsstörung. Während der Infusion verschlechtert sich die kardiale Situation (Arrhythmien und Kammertachykardie). Der unmittelbar nach Abbruch der Infusion bestimmte Theophyllin-Plasmakonzentrationswert (TSK) betrug 72,1 mg $\cdot$ l^{-1}. Eine nachträglich analysierte Probe, die bereits 7 Stunden vor Infusionsende abgenommen worden war, enthielt bereits 69,4 mg $\cdot$ l^{-1}. Aus weiterer TSK über 24 h konnte eine Abschätzung der Eliminationsleistung für Theophyllin erfolgen ($T_{1/2\,el}$ = 53,4 h). Der Zustand des Patienten verschlechtert sich am folgenden Tag akut; Tod unter den Zeichen des Linksherzversagens; terminaler Transaminasenanstieg, pathologisch-anatomisch ausgedehnter Vorder- und Hinterwandinfarkt, Aortenaneurysma.

Epikritisch zeigt dieser Verlauf folgende Merkmale:

— hohes Alter
— akute schwere Erkrankung mit Indikation für Theophyllin
— unvollständige Krankheits- und Medikamentenanamnese

76

— unerwartete Verschlechterung oder Zusatzsymptomatik
— hohe Theophyllin-Serumkonzentration
— extreme Verzögerung der Theophyllin-Elimination.

In verschiedenen Studien (z. B. [3—7]) wird bei älteren Patienten eine direkte und ausschließliche Altersabhängigkeit der Theophyllin-Elimination für unwahrscheinlich ange-

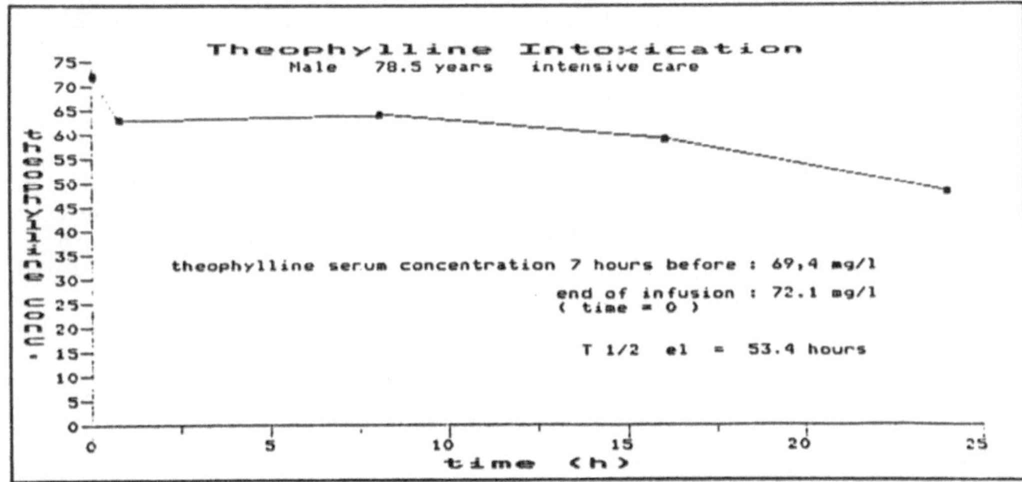

Abb. 1

Verlauf der Theophyllin-Serumkonzentrationswerte bei einem 78-jährigen Mann unter Intensivtherapie, präklinische Theophyllinmedikation unbekannt.

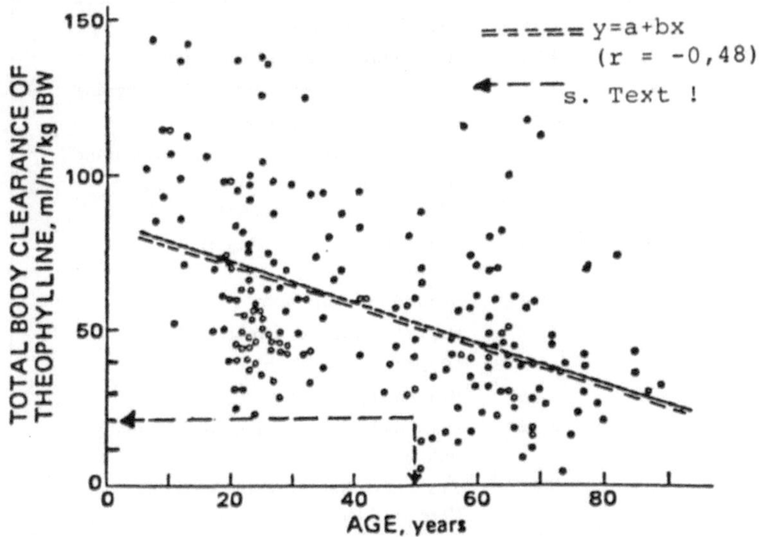

Abb. 2

Theophyllin-Clearancewerte von 200 Patienten und Freiwilligen, aufgetragen gegen das Lebensalter (aus [9], modifiziert).

sehen. Da in allen Altersstufen die Variabilität der Theophyllin-Clearance erheblich ist, könnte überhaupt nur an einem größeren Material ein statistischer Zusammenhang zwischen Lebensalter und Elimination sichtbar werden [8–10]. Die Analyse der JUSKO' Daten (Abb. 2, aus [9]) ergibt eine signifikant negative Korrelation zwischen Lebensalter und Theophyllin-Clearance, ferner ein ausschließliches Vorkommen von Clearance-Werten unter $20 \text{ ml} \cdot \text{h}^{-1} \cdot \text{kg}^{-1}$ jenseits des 50. Lebensjahres sowie statistisch eine Altersgrenze hinsichtlich verminderter Eliminationswerte beim 40. Lebensjahr. Dabei werden jenseits des 40. Jahres neben dem Alter als Einflußgrößen Leberschäden und kardiale Insuffizienz statistisch wirksam — ein Hinweis auf die multifaktorielle Konstellation der „Altersabhängigkeit" bei der Tendenz zur verminderten Elimination.

Dosisfindungsstudie bei über 65jährigen

Eine eigene Untersuchung umfaßt 12 Patienten jenseits des 65. Lebensjahres an einer kardiologischen Abteilung eines Kreiskrankenhauses. Bei diesen Patienten (Tabelle I) wurde vor einer beabsichtigten Theophyllin-Dauermedikation eine Testdosis einer Theophyllinlösung (Solldosis $4{,}5 \text{ mg} \cdot \text{kg}^{-1}$) zur individuellen Dosisfindung bei bekannter eliminationsbeeinflussender Grunderkrankung verabreicht.

Tabelle I Patientendaten, Diagnosen, Theophyllin-Testdosen.
* nach Frühstück; ** Abkürzungen: HI = Herzinsuffizienz, AVK = arterielle Verschlußkrankheit, TIA = transitorische ischämische Attacken; # und x s. Text.

Patient (Init./Geschlecht)		Alter (Jahre)	Gewicht (kg)	Dosis $(\text{mg} \cdot \text{kg}^{-1})$	Diagnosen **
1. E. D.	w	80	47	4,58	Oxazepam-Abusus
2. M. W.#	w	84	67	4,21	HI, cerebrovaskuläre Insuffizienz
3. E. S.	w	82	40	4,6	HI, Anämie, Cystenniere, AVK (Gangrän)
4. A. BD.	w	67	59	4,32	Diab. mell., Hemiparese, TIA
5. E. B.	w	83	58	4,37	Diab. mell., HI mit absoluter Arrhythmie
6. A. L. x	w	81	71	4,3	HI (Rekompensationsphase), Lungenödem, Niereninsuffizienz)
7. K.	m	72	66	4,54	M. Parkinson, Carotisstenose, Emphysem, multiple cerebrale Insulte
8. N. E.	m	85	50	4,24	Schilddrüsenkarzinom
9. P. P.	m	88	80	4,22	HI, Lebercirrhose, cerebraler Insult (Rekompensationsphase)
10. E. S.	m	79	62	4,36*	Bronchialkarzinom
11. W. L.	m	80	88	4,54*	Diab. mell., Hypertonie, Polyglobulie unklarer Genese
12. H. K.	m	89	68	4,27*	Zustand n. Herpes zoster N.trig. I li., Cerebralsklerose, Hyperurikämie

Untersuchungsbedingungen

— Keine Theophyllinmedikation während des bisherigen Klinikaufenthaltes
— Nahrungskarenz 12 Stunden (Ausnahmen: 3 männl. Patienten, in Tab. I mit * gekennzeichnet)
— „Methylxanthinkarenz" 12 Stunden (Einnahme sog. koffeinfreien Instant-Kaffees
wurde aus organisatorischen Gründen nicht ausgeschlossen)
— erste Nahrungsaufnahme 2 Stunden nach der Testdosis
— Probennahme 0.08; 0.16; 0.32; 0.66; 1; 2; 4; 6; 8; 12 und 24 Stunden nach der Testdosis, TSK-Bestimmung mittels HPLC entsprechend [11, 12].

Die TSK-Verläufe (Abb. 3) wurden zur Schätzung der Absorptions- und Eliminations-
Halbwertszeit (Regressionsgeraden des initialen und terminalen Konzentrations-Zeitver-
laufs; in geeigneten Fällen Absorptionshalbwertszeit nach Nelson und Wagner analog [11]),
des Verteilungskoeffizienten (C_0/Dosis) und der totalen Clearance verwendet und daraus
die Tagesdosis Theophyllin für eine Zielkonzentration von 15 mg/l bei den jeweiligen
Patienten berechnet.

Ergebnisse

Die kinetischen Parameter (Tabelle II) liegen mit einer Ausnahme (Patientin A. L. in
Tabelle I) im Bereich jüngerer Erwachsener.
Aus den Eliminationsparametern errechneten sich Tagesdosen zwischen 123 und 2852 mg
Theophyllin oder, auf das Körpergewicht bezogen, zwischen 1,73 und 46 mg·kg^{-1} (Tabel-
le III).

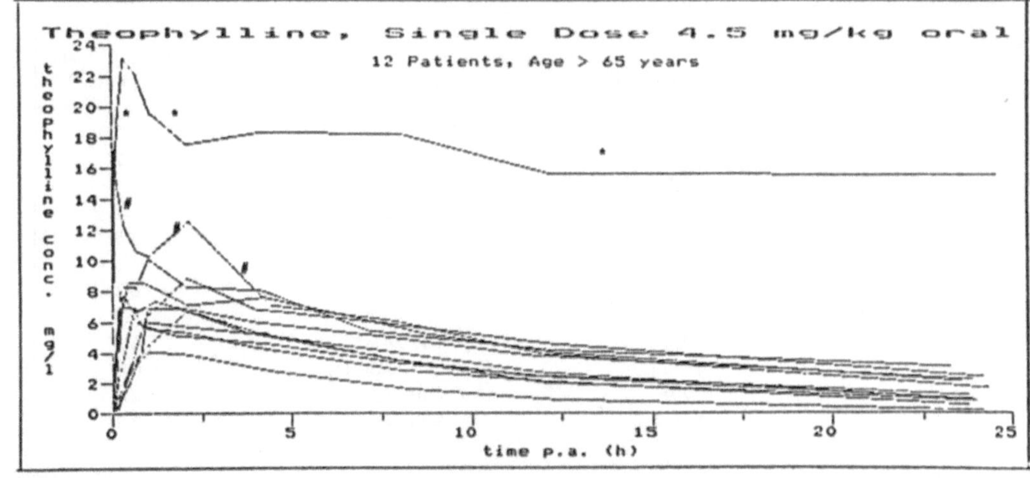

Abb. 3

Theophyllinkonzentrationsverläufe bei 12 über 65-jährigen nach einer Theophyllin-Testdosis von
4,0–4,5 mg · kg^{-1} oral; * A.L., # M.W. in Tabellen I und II, Einzelheiten im Text.

Tabelle II Pharmakokinetische Parameter von 12 Patienten > 65 Jahre:
c_{max} $(mg \cdot l^{-1})$, t_{max} (h), $AUC_{0 \to \infty}$ $(mg \cdot h \cdot kg^{-1}$, normiert auf $4{,}0\ mg \cdot kg^{-1})$, V_d $(l \cdot kg^{-1})$, $T_{1/2a}$ (h) (aus initialem Kurvenverlauf, in ( ) ggf. nach Nelson und Wagner errechnete Absorptionshalbwertszeit), $T_{1/2el}$ (h); weitere Details Tab. I.

Patient	c_{max}	t_{max}	AUC	V_d	$T_{1/2a}$	$T_{1/2el}$
1.	7,8	0,33	58,6	0,59	0,06 (0,18)	7,03
2.#	17,3	0,1	136,1	0,36	0,031	8,28
3.	7,0	0,61	55,8	0,74	0,11	6,57
4.	7,0	0,33	79,7	0,61	< 0,16	8,17
5.	10,1	1,0	163,8	0,47	< 0,16 (1,5)	13,4
6. x	(?)	0,35	(?)	0,48 (?)	0,31	69,8
7.	8,6	0,47	128,1	0,54	0,13 (0,06)	11,3
8.	6,7	2,0	74,5	0,57	0,31 (0,55)	7,7
9.	6,9	1,0	133,2	0,58	0,57 (0,2)	13,5
10.	4,1	1,0	31,5	0,84	0,3 (0,43)*	4,5
11.	8,9	2,0	123,0	0,5	0,19 (0,57)*	12,6
12.	7,6	0,25	81,7	0,72	0,15*	10,1

Tabelle III Theophyllin-Tagesdosen $(mg \cdot kg^{-1})$
errechnet für eine Serumkonzentration von $15\ mg \cdot l^{-1}$ bei einer angenommenen Bioverfügbarkeit = 100 %; * für täglich zweimalige Verabreichung und Verordnung üblicher Dosierungseinheiten von Theophyllin-Retardpräparaten; ** Zeit für steady state-Einstellung in Tagen.

Patient	kalkulierte Dosis		$15\ mg \cdot l^{-1}$ als C_{ss} nach **
	$mg \cdot kg^{-1} \cdot 24\ h^{-1}$	Einzeldosis*	
1.	20,85	500	1,5
2.#	10,85	350−375	1,7
3.	26,58	500	1,4
4.	18,49	500	1,7
5.	8,91	250	2,8
6. x	1,73 (!)	60 (!)	14,5 (!)
7.	11,9	400	2,4
8.	18,6	500	1,6
9.	10,6	400−450	2,8
10.	46,0 (!)	1400 (!)	0,9
11.	9,9	400−450	2,6
12.	17,6	500−600	2,1

Diskussion der Ergebnisse und Schlußfolgerungen

Die Variabilität der Eliminationsleistung bedingt in unserem Patientengut ein durchschnittliches Dosisverhältnis (Tagesdosis; $mg \cdot kg^{-1}$) von 1 : 3 ohne Extremwerte, einschließlich der beiden Extremfälle aber von fast 1 : 27. Für die Praxis der Therapie wichtig ist die Umrechnung auf die erforderlichen Dosierungen pro Einzelgabe, deren Verhältnis maximal ebenfalls 1 : 23 beträgt. Ohne die Extremfälle liegen andererseits die Einzeldosen für die erwünschte Konzentration im steady state ($C_{ss} = 15$ $mg \cdot l^{-1}$) bei dem für die Dauertherapie zweckmäßigsten Dosierungsintervall von 12 Stunden auch für die älteren Patienten höher (bei 8 Patienten bei 2 $\times$ 400 bis 500 mg) als heute allgemein klinisch üblich (2 $\times$ 250 bis 350 mg pro Tag). Das bestätigt die von uns allgemein für Erwachsene vertretene These, daß die heute übliche Routinedosierung von Theophyllin eine Ausschöpfung der Wirkungsreserven der Substanz verhindert [14, 15].

Der Medianwert des Verteilungskoeffizienten beträgt x = 0,585, der Mittelwert (= 0,58) weist einen VC = 22,1 % auf, die Extremwerte betragen 0,36 und 0,84 $l \cdot kg^{-1}$. Diese Werte sprechen gegen die Verallgemeinerungsfähigkeit der Schlußfolgerungen von ANTAL et al. [13], wonach für ältere Patienten ein größeres Risiko besonders bei Infusionsbehandlungen besteht, welches aus deren kleinerem Verteilungsvolumen infolge des höheren Anteils an freiem Theophyllin (Abb. 4, aus [13]) resultieren soll. In unserem Material fand sich lediglich bei einer Patienten (M. W. in Tab. II in Abb. 3 mit # gekennzeichnet) mit einem V_d von 0,36 ein über diesen Mechanismus erklärbarer Peakwert von 17,3 $mg \cdot l^{-1}$.

Dieses bei rigider Dosierung prinzipiell mögliche Risiko wird unseres Erachtens übertroffen von der ebenso wie bei jüngeren Personen vorhandenen Variabilität der Elimination. Besonders deutlich wird das bei den auch in unserem kleinen Untersuchungsmaterial vorhandenen „kritischen" Fällen (akute Verschlechterung der Grundkrankheit, akute Infektion, unbekannte Begleiterkrankung, Vormedikation u. a. Faktoren):

Typisch hierfür ist der Konzentrationsverlauf bei einer 81jährigen Patientin (A. L. in Tab. II, in Abb. 3 mit x gekennzeichnet): Diese befand sich zum Zeitpunkt der Testdosisverabreichung bereits eine Woche in der Klinik, von einer Theophyllinbehandlung war anamnestisch nichts bekannt. Sie erhielt wegen einer kardialen Dekompensation Metildigoxin, ein Furosemid-Canrenoat-Mischpräparat und Heparin. Der Theophyllinleerwert im Plasma betrug 10,3 $mg \cdot l^{-1}$, ferner wurde in allen Plasmaproben ein konstanter Koffeinwert von 3,1 $mg \cdot l^{-1}$ gemessen; der nach der Testdosis resultierende Theophyllin-Peakwert betrug 23,3 $mg \cdot l^{-1}$. Die Analogie zu dem oben dargestellten Intoxikationsfall ist offenkundig.

Die Variabilität der Therapievoraussetzungen besonders bei älteren Patienten erfordert zwingend eine an klinischer Wirkung und Serumkonzentration orientierte Dosierungskontrolle, sie verbietet eine unkontrollierte Routinedosierung von Theophyllinpräparaten (Dauermedikation oder Infusionstherapie) und schließt eine deduktive Dosisanpassung aufgrund allgemeiner Kriterien (z. B. hohes Alter, kardiale Dekompensation, interkurrente Erkrankung u. a.) aus, wie bereits aus anderen Untersuchungen unter Praxisbedingungen [14, 15] hervorgeht.

Eine Untersuchung von WESTERFIELD et al. [16] an 20 älteren Patienten einer Intensivstation konnte eine Tendenz zur „Abhängigkeit" der Theophyllin-Clearance vom klinischen Zustand nur tendenziell, nicht aber statistisch sichern. Es war auch keine Korrelation mit anderen bei der Schwere der Erkrankung häufig veränderten typischen Laborparametern (pH, p_aO_2, p_aCO_2) nachweisbar.

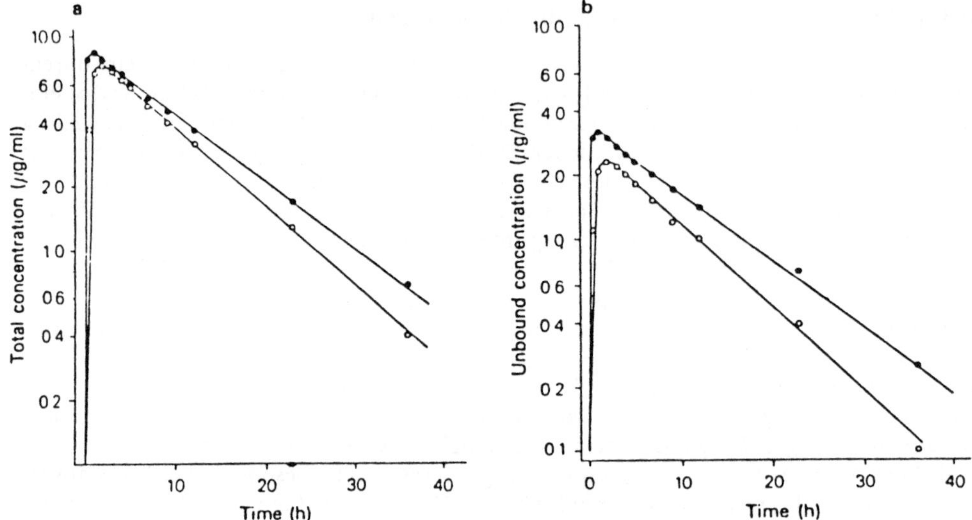

Mean semilogarithmic total (a) and unbound (b) plasma level-time profiles in elderly (●) and young (○) volunteers following a single 200 mg oral dose of theophylline.

Pharmacokinetic parameters derived from unchanged plasma theophylline ($\bar{x} \pm$ SD)

	N = 14 Control	N = 14 Elderly	
$T_{1/2}$ (h)	8.51 ± 2.00	9.81 ± 4.10	NS
V_d total (l/kg)	0.43 ± 0.06	0.32 ± 0.05	NS
$V_{d\,unbound}$ (l/kg)	1.38 ± 0.23	0.86 ± 0.14	$P < 0.005$
Total plasma clearance (ml/min)	34.9 ± 12.0	29.4 ± 9.99	NS
Unbound plasma clearance (ml/min)	113.5 ± 39.5	79.8 ± 29.7	$P < 0.02$

Abb. 4

Unterschiede pharmakokinetischer Parameter von Theophyllin bei je 14 jüngeren und älteren Erwachsenen [13]. Oberer Teil: Gesamt-Theophyllinkonzentration a) und Konzentration des freien Theophyllins b) für Personen von durchschnitt 23,1 ○ bzw. 76,2 ● Jahren.

Es ist also festzuhalten, daß die Ursachen der inter- und intraindividuellen Variabilität des Theophyllin-Metabolismus und deren Altersabhängigkeit bisher nicht geklärt werden konnten. Durch konsequente serumkonzentrationsorientierte individuelle Dosierung können aber in allen diesen Fällen Wirksamkeits- und Verträglichkeitsprobleme weitgehend vermieden werden.

Für die Kooperation bei der Durchführung der Untersuchungen danken wir Herrn Prof. Dr. G. Bodem und den Mitarbeitern der I. Medizinischen Klinik des Kreiskrankenhauses Homburg v. d. H. (Hochtaunuskreis) herzlich.

Literatur:

[1] *Hirsch, S.:* Klinischer und experimenteller Beitrag zur krampflösenden Wirkung der Purinderivate. Klin. Wschr. **1**, 615–618 (1923)

[2] *Herrmann, G., M. B. Aynesworth:* Successful treatment of persistent extrem dyspnea "status asthmaticus". J. Lab. Clin. Med. **23**, 135–148 (1937)

[3] *Nielsen-Kudsk, F., I. Magnussen, P. Jakobsen:* Pharmacokinetics of theophylline in ten elderly patients. Acta pharmacol. et toxicol. **42**, 226–234 (1978)

[4] *Piafsky, K. M., D. S. Sitar, R. E. Ragno, R. I. Ogilvie:* Theophylline Disposition in patients with hepatic cirrhosis. N. Engl. J. Med. **296**, 1495 (1977)

[5] *Powell, J. R., S. Vozeh, P. Hopewell, J. Costello, L. B. Sheiner, S. Riegelman:* Theophylline disposition in acutely ill hospitalized patients. The effect of smoking, heart failure, severe airway obstruction, and pneumonia. Am. Rev. Respir. Dis. **118**, 228–238 (1978)

[6] *Blaive, B., P. Lapalus, F. Lemoigne, B. Bugnas:* Theophylline: Parametres pharmacocinetiques et determination d'une posologie individuelle efficace. Bull. europ. Physiopath. **17**, 333–339 (1981)

[7] *Cusak, B., J. G. Kelly, J. Lavan, N. Noel, K. O'Malley:* The effect of age and smoking on theophylline kinetics. Br. J. Clin. Pharmac. **12**, 637–645 (1981)

[8] *Ogilvie, R. I.:* Clinical pharmacokinetics of theophylline. Clinical Pharmacokinetics **3**, 267–293 (1978)

[9] *Jusko, W. J., M. J. Gardner, A. Mangione, J. J. Schentag, J. R. Koup, J. W. Vance.* Factors effecting theophylline clearances: Age, tobacco, marijuana, cirrhosis, congistive heart failure, obesity, oral contraceptives, benzodiazeoines, barbiturates, and ethanol. J. Pharmaceut. Sci. **68**, 1358–1366 (1979)

[10] *Staib, A. H., H. H. Klemme, N. Heinz:* Variabilität der Theophyllinplasmakonzentration – retrospektive Studie über drei Jahre Drug Monitoring. In: Theophylline an other Methylxanthines. The Proceedings of an International Symposium Frankfurt 29th and 30th May 1981 (ed. *N. Rietbrock, B. G. Woodcock, A. H. Staib*) Vieweg-Verlag Braunschweig/Wiesbaden (1982), S. 273–281.

[11] *Staib, A. H., D. Loew, S. Harder, E. H. Graul, R. Pfab, B. Hugemann:* Theophylline absorption at different gastrintestinal sites in the man: Studies employing a remote control liberation system (HF-Capsule). Arch. Pharmacol. Suppl. **330**, R 15, abstract 66 (1985)

[12] *Caldwell, J., A. H. Staib, I. A. Cotgreave, M. Siebert-Weigel:* Intraindividual comparison of theophylline pharmacokinetics in human volunteers after intravenous infusion with ethylenediamine od sodium glycinate. Br. J. Clin. Pharmacol.: **22**, 351–355 (1968)

[13] *Antal, E. J., P. A. Kramer, S. A. Mercik, D. J. Chapron, I. R. Lawson:* Theophylline pharmacokinetics in advanced age. Br. J. Clin. Pharmac. **12**, 637–645 (1981)

[14] *Staib, A. H., N. Rietbrock, A. Neiss:* Bestimmung der Serum-Theophyllinkonzentration in der ambulanten Praxis. Dtsch. med. Wschr. **110**, 680–685 (1985)

[15] *Staib, A. H., J. Stauder, S. Harder:* Theophyllinmonitoring bei ambulanten Patienten. In: Drug Monitoring-Erfassung von Arzneimittelnebenwirkungen und Serumkonzentrationsbestimmungen von Pharmaka (ed. *H. Rameis, H. G. Hitzenberger*), 11. Symposium der Österreichischen Arbeitsgemeinschaft für Klinische Pharmakologie Wien 1983, Uhlen-Verlagsgesellschaft Wien (1984), S. 141–156

[16] *Westerfield, B. T., A. J. Carder, R. W. Light:* The relationship between arterial blood gases and serum theophylline clearance in critically ill patients. Am. Rev. Respir. Dis. **124**, 17–20 (1981)

New Aspects on Digitalis, the Drug of the Aged

B. G. Woodcock/N. Rietbrock
Abteilung für Klinische Pharmakologie, Universitätsklinik, Theodor-Stern-Kai 7,
6000 Frankfurt am Main 70.

Summary

Since the time of Withering, digitalis has been mainly used in the aged. Apart from patients with atrial fibrillation, those who are likely to benefit most from the drug are those who need an enhanced cardiac reserve. The presence of a third heart sound gallop on placebo, severe chronic rather than episodic congestive heart failure, marked ventricular dilatation and a decreased ejection fraction are characteristics of such patients. In about 30 % of cases the response to digitalis may be dramatic.
The elderly show an increased sensitivity to digitalis and about 20 % of patients admitted to medical wards will show some form of ECG-abnormality despite having a serum digitalis concentration in or even below the so-called therapeutic range. It follows that the commonly used method of administering a loading-dose to quickly attain a pre-chosen concentration in the therapeutic range is less suitable for elderly subjects. A safer approach is to begin therapy with a maintenance dose of digitoxin and monitor at weekly intervals for the first 2 or 3 weeks and then every 2 weeks building up to regular patient check-ups at 2 to 3 monthly intervals. Digoxin treatment in the elderly could also be started without a loading dose. Kinetic considerations dictate that initial monitoring (of the response, not the concentration) every 2 days building up to a monitoring frequency of once every 2 to 3 weeks is necessary. Less frequent monitoring will certainly put the patient at risk although the necessary controlled double blind studies to prove this unequivocally are not available. It is worthwhile remembering that subjective complaints of toxicity such as nausea and gastric disturbances, found useful in the past as warning symptoms of toxicity, may not be prominant in the elderly despite the appearance of ventricular arrhythmias and conduction abnormalities in the ECG.

Zusammenfassung

Seit Withering wird Digitalis hauptsächlich beim älteren Patienten verordnet. Neben Patienten mit Vorhofflimmern profitieren besonders Patienten mit drittem Herzton, ventrikulärer Dilatation, reduziertem Cardiac Index und mit chronischer, nichtepisodischer Herzinsuffizienz von der Therapie. In 30 % der Fälle sprechen diese Patienten auf die Therapie sofort an.
Ältere Patienten reagieren empfindlicher auf Digitalis, so daß 20 % der unter ärztlicher Aufsicht stehenden Patienten trotz Digitalis-Serumkonzentrationen im oder unter dem therapeutischen Bereich Veränderungen im EKG aufweisen. Subjektive

Klagen über Nebenwirkungen wie Nausea und Magenbeschwerden, die in der Vergangenheit als wichtige Symptome für eine beginnende Intoxikation galten, treten im Alter nicht so häufig auf, obwohl ventrikuläre Arrhythmien und Überleitungsstörungen im EKG beobachtet werden. Daraus folgt, daß die übliche „loading dose" zum schnellen Erreichen einer „steady state" Konzentration ungeeignet ist. Ein sicherer Ansatz wäre, mit der Erhaltungsdosis von Digitoxin zu beginnen. In den ersten 2-3 Wochen sollte der Therapieerfolg wöchentlich, dann in Abständen von 2 Wochen kontrolliert werden. In der späteren Langzeittherapie genügt die Überprüfung im 2-3 monatigen Abstand. Die Behandlung des älteren Patienten mit Digoxin sollte ebenfalls ohne „loading dose" beginnen. Die Pharmakokinetik des Digoxin verlangt, bei Beginn der Therapie weniger die Serumkonzentration als die Rekompensationszeichen des Patienten im Abstand von 2-3 Tagen zu beobachten. Spätere Kontrollen sind alle 2-3 Wochen notwendig. Die weniger häufige Kontrolle setzt den Patienten vermutlich einem erhöhten Risiko aus. Doppelblind-Studien, die dies eindeutig beweisen könnten, liegen aber nicht vor.

Digitalis: Mainly a Drug of the Aged

The average age of patients treated with digitalis by William Withering up to 1785 was between 40 and 50 years (Fig. 1) [2]. 200 years later, the age distribution of the patients receiving basically the same drug and for the same or similar indications has been displaced upwards by about 25 years. This shift is presumably due to general improvements in health and increase in longevity as illustrated for patients treated in the University Clinic Frankfurt (Fig. 2). Digitalis is therefore a drug used predominantly in the aged.

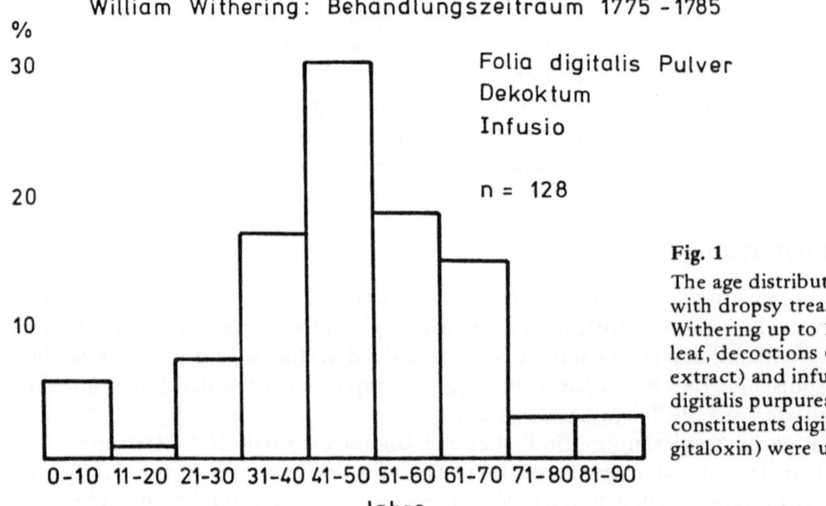

Fig. 1
The age distribution of patients with dropsy treated by William Withering up to 1785. Powdered leaf, decoctions (boiled aqueous extract) and infusions of digitalis purpurea (active constituents digitoxin and gitaloxin) were used.

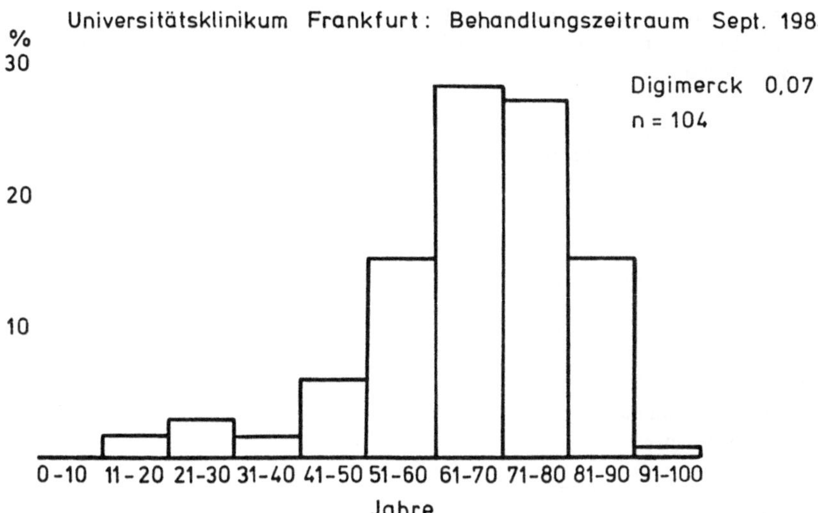

Fig. 2

Age distribution of in-patients of the University Clinic Frankfurt who were being treated with digitoxin between January 1984 and September 1984.

When to start Treatment

Digitalis is a good choice as first drug in patients with congestive heart failure or atrial
fibrillation and a rapid ventricular response. Recent studies describe the effect of discontinuing digitalis treatment during prolonged therapy where many patients were found to
manage just as well off the drug as on it with no worsening of the symptoms (Boman
et al. 1983 [1], Keller et al. this volume). In some patients it appeared that digitalis therapy
had been started without a sound indication. There is difficulty in identifying patients
with congestive heart failure and sinus rhythm in whom the drug will be effective and
where the benefits outweigh the hazards.

Improving Cardiac Efficiency

After attention to underlying causes such as hypertension or endocarditis (Table I) the
pharmacotherapy of congestive heart failure is commonly considered under 3 categories
according to the potential for.
1) an improvement of pumping performance with digitalis
2) the reduction of cardiac workload with vasodilators
3) reduction of cardiac workload through control of excessive salt and water retention
   with diuretics.

The mechanism by which each of these drugs alleviates congestive symptoms is shown in a plot of left ventricular end diastolic pressure against stroke volume (Fig. 3). Patients with depressed left ventricular performance and low output syndrome with increased filling pressure should benefit from diuretic therapy, with a shifting of the patients condition along the lower curve.

Table I: Underlying causes of heart failure

Underlying causes of heart failure

Surgical

congenital and acquired abnormalities

Medical

infectious endocarditis, hypertension

Precipitating causes

anaemia, rhythm disturbances, pulmonary emboli, coronary flow disturbances, hyperthyroid states

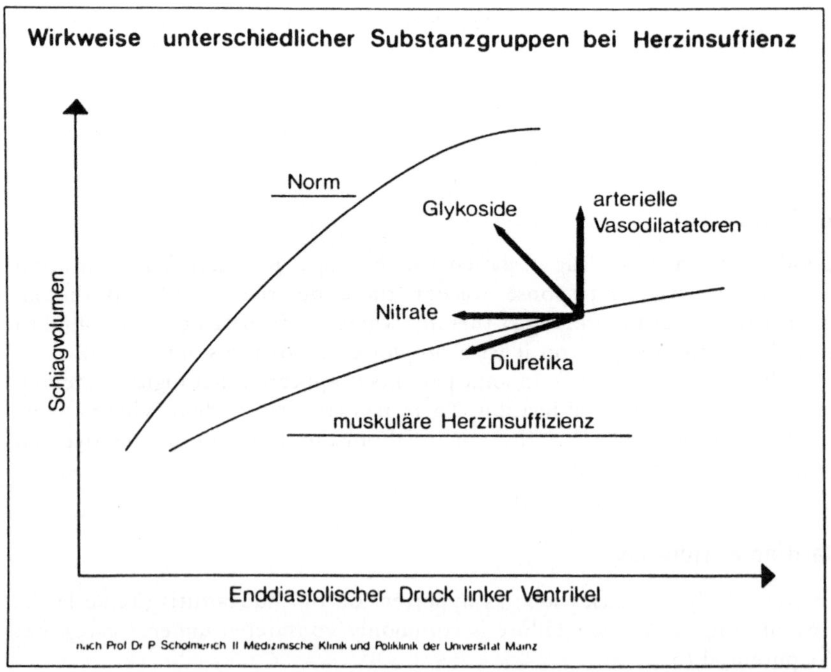

Fig. 3
This plot of left ventricular end diastolic pressure and stroke volume shows the reduction occurring during cardiac insufficiency and how cardiac glycosides, diuretic drugs and vasodilators can improve this function equation.

Patients who do not achieve a satisfactory response to judicious use of diuretics alone and who would benefit from enhanced cardiac reserve are the group who are likely to benefit from digitalis in order to shift the entire curve towards normal.

Lee, Johnson and Bingham et al. (1982) [5] have examined the criteria helpful in identifiying those subjects with cardiac insufficiency in sinus rhythm who are likely to improve on digitalis.

In this placebo controlled, randomised, crossover study, the 25 ambulatory patients, aged between 40 and 83 years (60 % classified as elderly according to the FDA criteria), all had congestive heart failure according to symptoms including x-ray and in some cases invasive tests, and all were receiving digixon and nearly all were on diuretics, mostly furosemide and 6 were receiving additional vasodilator therapy. In one of the two double-blind comparison periods serum digoxin concentrations in the range 1.2 to 1.4 ng/ml were aimed for and placebo was applied during the other comparison period.

The global insufficiency score was reduced from 3.6 to 2.7 by digitalis. 15 Patients showed a positive response and in 5 patients this was dramatic. 11 patients showed no apparent benefit but a closer inspection of these 11 patients throws much light on the criteria which may be useful for future identification of subgroups. 7 of the 11 had a heart failure score of zero on placebo, i.e. they were unable to show a response to digitalis at the time of the study using the score system employed and were well compensated on diuretics. 4 of the 11 patients had hypertrophic cardiomyopathy with ejection fractions greater than 50 % and would not be suitable candidates for digitalis except in the context of accompanying atrial fibrillation. 2 of the 11 paients had ischemic heart disease and ejection fractions greater than 60 %. Improvement here would not be expected since systolic function is adequate. 3 of the 11 patients had serum digoxin concentrations of 0.5 ng/ml which is probably at the threshold of the positive inotropic response to digoxin.

In summary, allowing for the 4 hypertrophic cardiomyopathy patients, the 2 with ischemic heart disease and 3 with low concentrations, 14 of the remaining 16 patients actually improved. These patients were characterised by the following:

1. All had a 3rd heart sound gallop on placebo
2. CHF was more severe and chronic rather than episodic
3. ejection fraction decrease and left ventricular dilatation was greater than in the other patients

In conclusion, patients with dilated ventricles and poor systolic function are most likely to benefit among the large group of patients with symptoms suggesting CHF with sinus rhythm. This study provided therefore much needed data on subjective as well as objective responses of ambulatory patients with reasonably well defined signs and symptoms of heart failure. However it still does not answer the question which patients will have a favourable risk-benefit ratio or which dose of digitalis will be most suitable (Smith, 1985 [6]).

The Choice of Cardiac Glycoside in the Aged

When one examines the prescribing habits of different countries one sees that the choice of glycoside is based on custom or habit rather than rational appraisal. Most clinicians are aware however that there are at least two types of glycosides for oral maintenance therapy, namely digoxin and digitoxin. The former has low serum protein binding and predominantly renal elimination, the other being highly bound in serum and cleared by renal and extra-renal routes.

Table II: True end-organ sensitivity to toxic effects of digitalis

Advanced myocardial disease
Active myocardial ischaemia
Hypokalaemina
Acid base imbalance
Concomitant drug administration (eg catecholamines)
Hypothyroidism
Hypoxia (especially acute respiratory failure)
Altered autonomic tone (vagotonic states)

Pharmacodynamic considerations: Elderly patients with chronic severe cardiac insufficiency have an increased susceptibility to the toxic effects of digitalis. There is for example an increased prevelance of ventricular ectopy accompanying the increase in age and organic heart disease. Sonnenblick and Abraham (1985) [7] observed that 13 of 61 geriatric patients, (21 %), with CHF or AF and with low-to-normal serum digoxin concentrations (< 2.6 nmol/l digoxin) had ECG signs compatible with toxicity. The causes of true end-organ sensitivity to toxic effects of digitalis are listed in Table II. Landahl et al. (1977) [4] observed that the frequency of ventricular extrasytoles in the aged is greater when treated with digoxin in comparison with digitoxin. However, there is very limited information available in which the inherent toxicities of the two molecules have been compared and so a preference for one drug or the other on the basis of toxic properties cannot be made at the present time.

Pharmacokinetic considerations: Although digitoxin, and for example gitoformate and acetylgitoxin, have renal independent elimination, without doubt a major advantage in the elderly because of the lower and changing renal function, digoxin is more widely used. It is generally believed that the shorter halflife of digoxin and the ability to rapidly escape from toxicity justifies its use in the aged. This has been thought to reduce the threat to life.

Rapidly disappearing drugs however must be monitored more often. This reasoning, well known for nitroprusside, has been applied to analysis of digitalis therapy. Here too, just as it is good to get out of toxicity fast, it is bad to get into it fast (Fig. 4). Jelliffe (1983) [3] has calculated that digoxin accumulation is 8 times more rapid than digitoxin 1 day after a fall in creatine clearance from 100 to 75 ml/min, and even in uremic patients is more than 3-fold more rapid (Table III). In clinical terms, digitoxin has a much slower onset of toxicity and consequently earlier detection at equal observation frequency. This is an advantage additional to having a total body digitoxin clearance which is independent of the renal function.

References

[1] Boman, K.: Digoxin and the geriatric in-patient. Acta Med Scand, **214**, 353–60, 1983.
[2] Estes, J.W.: Hall Jackson and the purple foxglove. University Press of New England, 1979, New Hampshire, USA.
[3] Jelliffe, R.W.: Digitalis therapy: The case for digitoxin. Abstract C18, Amer. Soc. Clinical Pharmacology and Therapeutics. Clin. Pharm Ther. February 1983.
[4] Landahl, S., Lindblad, B., Roupe, S., Steen, B., Svanborg, A.: Digitalis therapy in a 70-year old population. Acta med. Scand., **202**, 437–443, 1977.

[5] Lee, D.C., Johnson, R., Bingham, J.B. et al: Heart failure in outpatients. N. Eng. J. Med., **306**, 699–705, 1982.

[6] Smith, T.W.: Role of digitalis in long-term management of cardiac failure with sinus rhythm. Hammersmith Cardiology Workshop Series (Ed. Manseri, A.) Vol. **2**, 151–160, 1985.

[7] Sonnenblick, M., Abraham, A.S.: Digoxin treatment and control in the elderly. Isreal J Med Sci., **21**, 276–278, 1985.

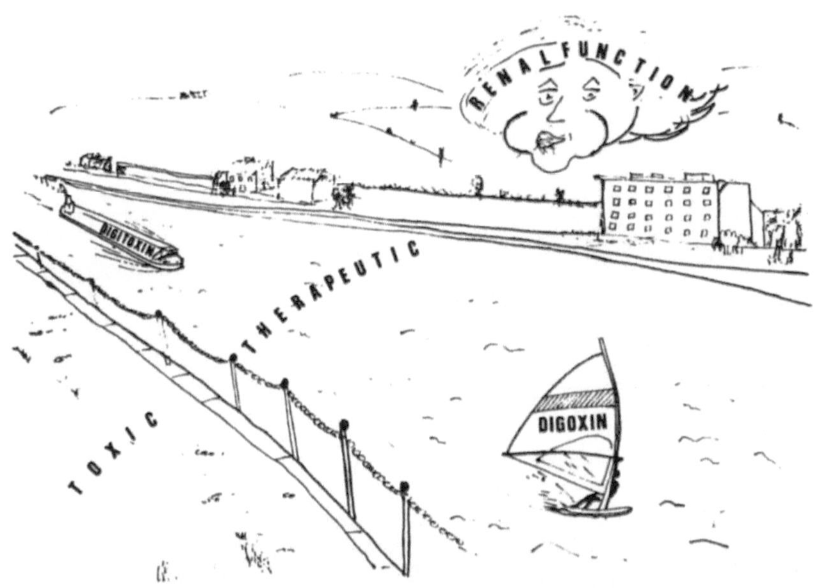

Fig. 4

This illustration is a 'nautical' interpretation of the concept of 'steerability' as applied to digitoxin and digoxin. Because of digoxin's rapid accumulation the drug response (position of the windsurfer) must be monitored 4 to 5 times as frequently as digitoxin, the barge, in order to detect the same change in course on the river. Thus the windsurfer must constantly attend to navigation. The problem of a decreased and sometimes varying renal function in aged patients is depicted here as the wind. The windsurfer must also make constant course corrections to take this into account. Conclusion: 'Windsurfing is for the young. The aged patient is much safer on the barge!'.

Table III: Accumulation rate of digoxin as a function of creatinine clearance

Change in Creatinine clearance (ml/min)	Accumulation rate of digoxin 1 day later. (Digitoxin = 1)
Fall from 100 to 75	8.4
Fall from 75 to 50	5.7
Fall from 50 to 25	3.9
Fall from 25 to 0	3.3

Halflife digoxin taken as 1.5 days
Halflife for digitoxin taken as 6 days

The Discontinuation of Digitalis Glycoside Therapy in the Elderly

F. Keller, D. Andresen, A. Schwarz, H.-F. Voehringer
Freie Universität, Klinikum Steglitz, Medizinische Klinik, Hindenburgdamm 30,
D-1000 Berlin 45,

Summary

Digitalis is the drug of the aged. Discontinuation of digitalis in selected patients is possible in 40 % to 100 % of the cases without a detrimental effect. After discontinuation of digitalis, atrial fibrillation and heart failure will occur in 5 % to 20 % of the cases. The use of digitoxin in hemodialysis patients does not increase the frequency of ventricular ectopic beats. The indications for digitalis treatment should be atrial fibrillation and heart failure and not the causes of heart failure per se (age, hypertension, coronary artery or valvular heart diesease, cardiomyopathy, uremia). The value of digitalis increases as heart failure progresses. Since heart failure advances with age, the "truth" appears to lie between the extremes: critical use but no rigorous withdrawal of digitalis glycosides in the elderly.

Key Words

Digoxin, Digitoxin, Aged, Hemodialysis, Arrhythmias

Introduction

Age is a risk factor for nearly every disease. In our population, 16 % are older than 65 years (Franke, 1983). A drug is prescribed to 72 % of all patients older than 65 years (Black, 1984). The risk of adverse drug effects increases from 5 % in all to 20 % in older patients (Black, 1984). Digitalis is the drug of the aged. Nearly 5 % of all West Germans receive digitalis (Schueren, 1982). Most are more than 65 years old where the percentage receiving digitalis approaches 41 % (Middeke, 1985). The rationale for this practice has been questioned in several studies, especially since the therapeutic range of cardiac glycosides is narrow.

Digitalis Discontinuation

Controlled studies on digitalis discontinuation showed that it is prescribed too often and often without sufficient reason. These studies date from 1970 to the present (Table I). Investigations were usually performed in outpatients but very often in geriatric patients as well in whom the various causes of heart failure were hypertension, coronary artery or valvular heart disease, cardiomypathy, uremia or old age. The size of groups investigated

Table I: Studies on discontinuation of digitalis glycoside therapy (1)

Author/Year	Patient group	Journal
Dall 1970	hospital/practice	Br. Med. J.
Hull 1977	practice	Lancet
Johnston 1979	outpatient	Lancet
Krakauer 1979	geriatric	Dan. Med. Bull.
Boman 1981	geriatric	Acta. Med. Scand.
Lee 1982	outpatient	N. Engl. J. Med.
Taggart 1983	outpatient	J. Cardiovasc. Pharm.
Gheorghiade 1983	coron. art. dis.	Am. J. Cardiol.
Boman 1983	geriatric	Acta. Med. Scand.
Keller 1984	hemodialysis	Dtsch. Med. Wschr.
Schüffler 1985	hospital	Z. Klin. Med.
Middeke 1985	outpatient	Klin. Wschr.

Discontinuation of digitalis glycoside therapy (2)

Author/Year	Number of patients	Observation period
Dall 1970	n = 80	3 months
Hull 1977	n = 24	3 months
Johnston 1979	n = 56	3 months
Krakauer 1979	n = 1854	2 months
Boman 1981	n = 141	2 months
Lee 1982	n = 25	12 months
Taggart 1983	n = 22	6 months
Gheorghiade 1983	n = 114	1 month
Boman 1983	n = 232	4 months
Keller 1984	n = 110	12 months
Schüffler 1985	n = 1699	1 month
Middeke 1985	n = 4143	3 months

Discontinuation of digitalis glycoside therapy (3)

Author/Year	Excluded because of Atrial fibrillation		Other cause	
Dall 1970	?		?	
Hull 1977	6/24	(25 %)	?	
Johnston 1979	?		?	
Krakauer 1979	22/82	(27 %)	32/54	(59 %)
Boman 1981	24/141	(17 %)	?	
Lee 1982	?		?	
Taggart 1983	?		?	
Gheorghiade 1983	26/114	(23 %)	90/114	(79 %)
Boman 1983	6/66	(9 %)	14/66	(21 %)
Keller 1984	10/110	(9 %)	5/110	(5 %)
Schüffler 1985			257/503	(51 %)
Middeke 1985	48/220	(22 %)	477/508	(94 %)

Discontinuation of digitalis glycoside therapy (4)

Author/Year	Withdrawal possible		Mean age of patients
Dall 1970	59/80	(74 %)	78 years (58-99)
Hull 1977	17/24	(71 %)	75 years (56-97)
Johnston 1979	48/56	(86 %)	65 years
Krakauer 1979	16/22	(73 %)	82 years (58-98)
Boman 1981	108/134	(81 %)	80 years (67-95)
Lee 1982	11/25	(44 %)	61 years (40-83)
Taggart 1983	16/22	(73 %)	65 years
Gheorghiade 1983	24/24	(100 %)	60 years (42-80)
Boman 1983	32/37	(86 %)	79 years (55-90)
Keller 1984	22/57	(39 %)	56 years (25-80)
Schüffler 1985	122/122	(100 %)	?
Middeke 1985	24/26	(92 %)	73 years (50-83)

Discontinuation of digitalis glycoside therapy (5)

Author/Year	Events Atrial fibrillation		Heart failure	
Dall 1970		(0 %)		(0 %)
Hull 1977	6/24	(25 %)	1/24	(4 %)
Johnston 1979	6/56	(11 %)	2/56	(4 %)
Krakauer 1979		(0 %)	5/22	(23 %)
Boman 1981	6/134	(4 %)	13/134	(10 %)
Lee 1982		(0 %)	14/25	(56 %)
Taggart 1983	1/22	(5 %)	6/22	(27 %)
Gheorghiade 1983		(0 %)		(0 %)
Boman 1983	5/39	(13 %)		(0 %)
Keller 1983	4/70	(6 %)	13/70	(19 %)
Schüffler 1985		(0 %)		(0 %)
Middeke 1985	2/26	(8 %)		(0 %)

ranged from 22 to 4143 patients and the observation period from 1 to 12 months. Approximately half of the patients were primarily excluded from withdrawal studies because of atrial fibrillation in up to 15 % of them, among various other reasons. Most patients were older than 65 years. Up to 50 % of all patients had a subtherapeutic digitalis plasma concentration (Middeke 1985). Discontinuation of digitalis was possible in 39 % to 100 % of the patients. Deterioration of heart failure after digitalis withdrawal occurred in 4 % to 27 % of the patients. The benefit of digitalis increased with advancing heart failure as indicated by a third heart sound (Lee 1982). Without digitalis atrial fibrillation became apparent in up to 25 % of the patients (Boman 1983).

Digitalis in Hemodialysis Patients

We have undertaken a digitalis withdrawal study in hemodialysis patients (Keller, 1984). Digitalis could not be discontinued because of atrial fibrillation in 10 and recurrent pulmonary edema in 5 of 110 hemodialysis patients (Fig. 1). Of the 70 patients investigated,

57 were on digitoxin, and in 22 of the 57 patients (39 %), digitoxin could be discontinued for 4 to 6 weeks without a detrimental effect. Digitoxin was given to 13 patients not yet on digitalis and had a beneficial effect in 3 of them (23 %). In 4 patients, atrial fibrillation occurred after discontinuation of digitoxin but in no patient on digitoxin (Fig. 2). The radiological signs of heart faiure deteriorated without digitoxin in 12 patients (Fig. 3). Uremia must be considered a particular cause of heart failure (Hung, 1980). The median

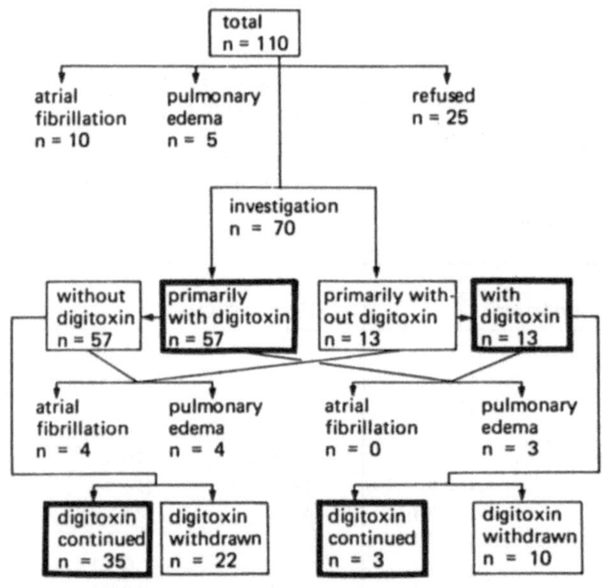

Fig. 1

Design of the digitalis discontinuation study in 110 hemodialysis patients.

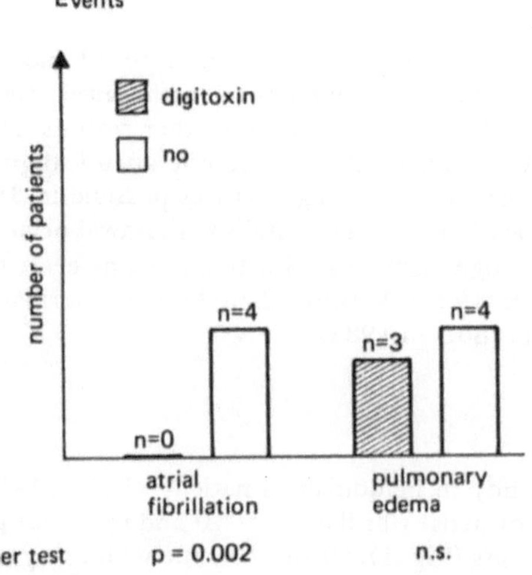

Fig. 2

After discontinuation of digitoxin, atrial fibrillation occurred in 4 patients. Occurrence of pulmonary edema was not significantly different.

age of patients who showed benefit from digitalis was 59 years; they were significantly older than those in whom digitoxin could be discontinued (Fig. 4). A digitoxin intoxication became clinically apparent in 3 % of the patients and was rare (Fig. 5). Also in the literature, the frequency of digitalis intoxication decreased from 20 % to less than 10 % within the

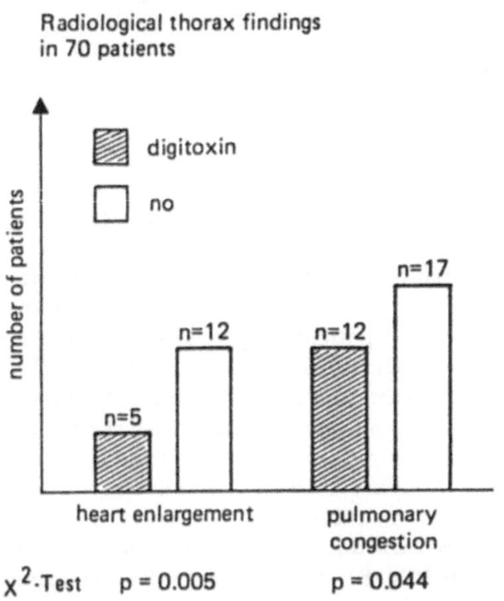

Fig. 3
Radiological thorax findings deteriorated in 12
patients after discontinuation of digitoxin.

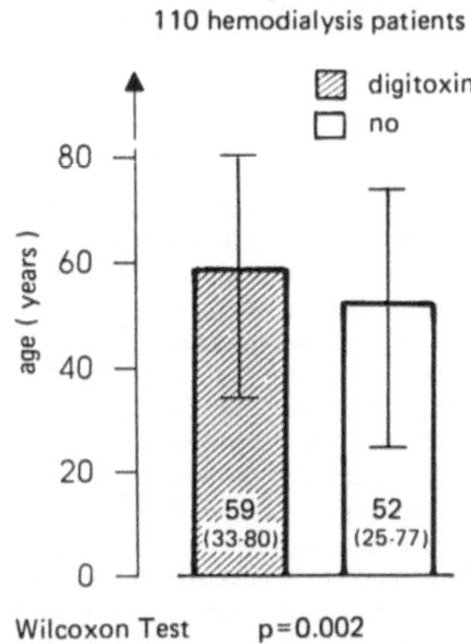

Fig. 4
Patients in whom digitalis treatment was
continued were significantly older than
those in whom no indication to digitalis
treatment was seen.

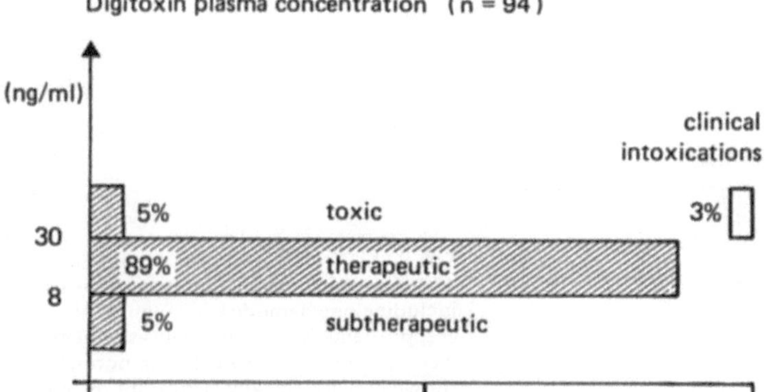

Fig. 5
Frequency of elevated digitoxin concentration was low, and clinically apparent digitalis intoxications
were rare within the 12-month observation period.

last 15 years (Smith, 1984). Our conclusion was that 57 % of the hemodialysis patients should be maintained on digitoxin. those with atrial fibrillation and those with signs of heart failure. This conclusion was vigorously doubted (Kramer, 1984). Digitoxin is supposed to induce arrhythmias on hemodialysis due to heparinization and decreased plasma protein binding. Thus digitalis may even be a dangerous drug. An objection to our study was that hypertension was in-adequately treated in 70 % of the patients. The term "malpractice" was even used. The occurrence of complex ventricular tachycardias leading to ventricular fibrillation was suspected to be the main risk and long-term electrocardiographic monitoring was recommended (Kramer, 1984).

Electrocardiographic Monitoring

We have already investigated this problem in our study and the preliminary results are presented here. In each hemodialysis patient, a 48-hour electrocardiographic monitoring, including one hemodialysis treatment, was carried out whilst on digitoxin, and 4 to 6 weeks after discontinuation of digitalis. In 50 % of the patients, no ventricular ectopic beats were seen. Complex ventricular actopic beats occurred in 13 patients (24 % without multiple counting). There was no difference with and without digitoxin (Fig. 6). Ventricular ectopic beats are also found in 45 % of healthy volunteers and even complex arrhythmias in 20 % of the cases (von Leitner 1983). The type of complex arrhythmias in the hemodialysis patients, showed no differences with or without digitoxin (Fig. 7). The frequency of ventricular ectopic beats on hemodialysis was higher than in the following hours. Statistically significant differences were only found on the second day when the mean frequency of ventricular ectopic beats in patients with digitoxin was even significantly **lower** than in the same patients without digitoxin (Fig. 8). An anamnestic hypertension was present in 74 % of all investigated patients but after commencement of hemodialysis treatement antihypertensive medication was required in only 34 % of the patients. This is no greater than in other dialysis centers (Kramer, 1984).

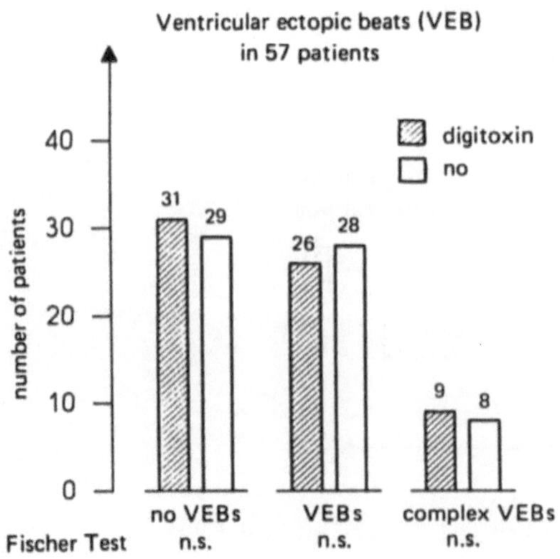

Fig. 6
48-hour electrocardiographic monitoring including one hemodialysis. Ventricular ectopic beats in 57 hemodialysis patients were not more frequent than in normals and showed no statistically significant differences with and without digitoxin.

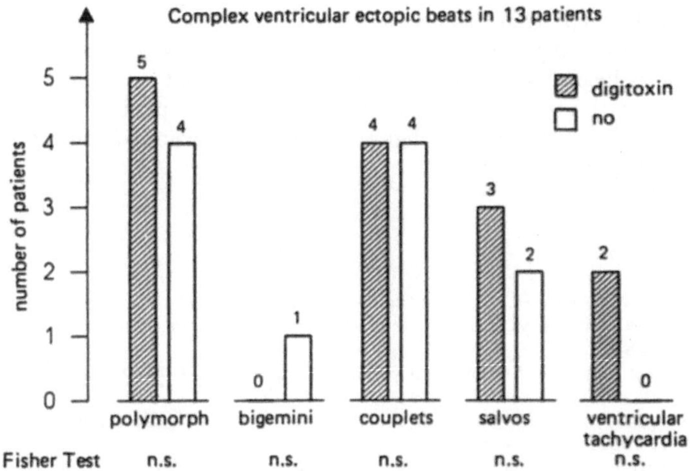

Fig. 7

Complex ventricular ectopic beats in 9 and 8 hemodialysis patients with and without digitoxin respectively. No statistically significant differences were found.

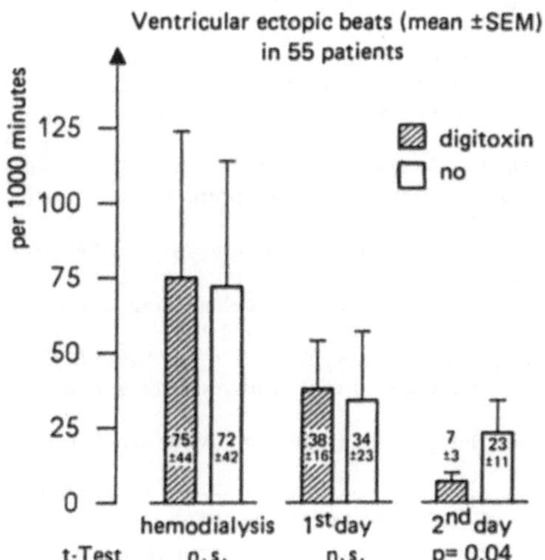

Fig. 8

Frequency of ventricular ectopic beats in 55 hemodialysis patients with and without digitoxin. On the day without hemodialysis (2nd day) ventricular ectopic beats were significantly less frequent with digitoxin than without.

Conclusions

The indication for digitalis treatment is atrial fibrillation (with tachyarrhythmia) and heart failure (Arnold, 1980/Weiner, 1983). The possible causes of heart failure alone do not sufficiently justify digitalis treatment (age, hypertension, coronary artery on valvular heart disease, cardiomyopathy and uremia). There is no doubt that digitalis is prescribed too frequently and often without good reason. The other extreme would be to withhold and withdraw digitalis. Thus the beneficial effects of digitalis would be lost as was just shown in the discontinuation studies. Digitalis may be withdrawn in patients without atrial fibrillation and without obvious heart failure or if neither can be affirmed by anamnesis. Digitalis can be withdrawn in patients with no symptoms and subtherapeutic digitalis levels. In doubt, however, especially in the elderly, digitalis should be continued, since the aged are often the diseased among us.

References

Arnold, S.B., Byrd, R.C. Meister, W., Melmon, K., Cheitlin, M.D., Bristow, J.D., Parmley, W.W., Chatterjee, K.: Long-term digitalis therapy improves left ventricular function in heart failure. N. Engl. J. Med. 303, 1443-8, 1980.

Black, D.: Medicatin for the elderly. A report of the royal college of physicians. J. Roy. Coll. Phys. Lond., 18, 7-17, 1984.

Boman, K., Allgulander, S., Skoglund, M.: Is maintenance digoxin necessary in geriatric patients? Acta. Med. Scand., 210, 493-5, 1981.

Boman, K.: Digoxin and the geriatric in-patient. Acta. Med. Scand., 214, 353-60, 1983.

Dall, J.L.C.: Maintenance digoxin in elderly patients. Br. Med. J. 1, 705-6, 1970.

Franke, H.: Einleitung und Einführung zur Gerotherapie. In (Ed.) *Franke, H.:* Gerotherapie. Fischer, Jena, 1, 1983.

Gheoghiade, M., Beller, G.A.: Effects of discontinuing maintenance digoxin therapy in patients with ischemic heart disease and congestive heart failure in sinus rhythm. Am. J. Cardiol., 51, 1243-50, 1983.

Hull, S.M., Mackintosh, A.: Discontinuation of maintenance digoxin therapy in general practice. Lancet 2, 1054-5, 1977.

Hung, J., Harris, P.J., Uren, R.F., Tiller, D.J., Kelly, D.T.: Uremic cardiomyopathy — effect of hemodialysis on left ventricular function in end-stage renal failure. N. Engl. J. Med., 302, 547-51, 1980.

Johnston, G.D., McDevitt, D.G.: Is maintenance digoxin necessary in patients with sinus rhythm? Lancet 1, 567-70, 1979.

Keller, F., Schwarz, A., Offermann, G., Molzahn, M., Distler, A., Kreutz, G., Weinmann, J., von Leitner, E.R., Voehringer, H.F.: Digitalis-Auslaßversuch bei Hämodialyse-Patienten. Deutsch. Med. Wochenschr. 109, 290-4, 1984.

Krakauer, R., Petersen, B.: The effects of discontinuing maintenance digoxin therapy; a study of elderly cardiac patients in sinus rhythm. Dan. Med. Bull. 26, 10-3, 1979.

Kramer, P., Girndt, J., Eisenhauer, T., Bethge, K.P., Wigger, W., Valentin, R.: Behandlung kardiovaskulärer Erkrankungen bei Dialysepatienten. Nieren Hochdruckkrh. 13, 271-94, 1984.

Lee, D.C.S., Johnson, R.A., Bingham, J.B., Leahy, M., Dinsmore, R.E., Goroll, A.H., Newell, J.B., Strauss, H.W., Haber, E.: Heart failure in outpatients. A randomized trial of digoxin versus placebo. N. Engl. J. Med. 306, 699-705, 1982.

Leitner von, E.R., Schröder, R.: Das Langzeit-EKG bei Herzgesunden. Deutsch. Med. Wochenschr. 108, 523-6, 1983.

Middeke, M., Meister, W., Krüger, C., Krahl, B., Holzgreve, H.: Digitalistherapie: Verschreibungshäufigkeit, Serumkonzentrationen und Auslaßversuch. Klin. Wochenschr. 63, 775-80, 1985.

Schüffler, J., Pense, G.: Nichtindizierte Digitalistherapie — ein Beitrag zur wissenschaftlich begründeten Arzneimittelverordnung. Z. Klin. Med. 40, 561-2, 1985.

Schüren, K.P., Rietbrock, N.: Digitalisbehandlung in Deutschland. Beispiel einer unkritischen Arzneimittelverordnung. Deutsch. Med. Wochenschr. 107, 1935-8, 1982.

Smith, T.W., Antman, E.M., Friedman, P.L., Blatt, C.M., Marsch, J.D.: Digitalis glycosides: mechanisms and manifestations of toxicity. Progr. Cardiovasc. Dis. 26, 413-58, 1984.

Taggart, A.J., Johnston, G.D., McDevitt, D.G.: Digoxin withdrawal after cardiac failure in patients with sinus rhythm. J. Cardiovasc. Pharmacol. 5, 229-34, 1983.

Weiner, P., Bassan, M.M., Jarchovsky, J., Iusim, S., Plavnick, L.: Clinical course of acute atrial fibrillation treated with rapid digitalization. Am. Heart. J. 105, 223-7, 1983.

Cytostatic Drug Treatment in the Elderly

H. Breithaupt
Medizinische Klinik I und II am Zentrum für Innere Medizin,
Klinikum der Justus-Liebig-Universität Gießen, Klinikstraße 36, 6300 Gießen, FRG.

Summary

The available knowledge on cytostatic drug treatment in the elderly is very scanty. An age dependent decrease in the renal clearance of the folate antoganist methotrexate has been shown. Metabolism and clearance of 5-fluorouracil, however, is not reduced in the aged. A dose reduction for 6-thioguanine, 6-mercaptopurine, or azathioprine may be necessary in the elderly. Infusion of high doses of cytarabin is followed by significantly higher plasma concentrations of the uracil-metabolite in elderly patients, presumably due to delayed renal excretion. No dose adjustment is necessary in the elderly treated with cyclophosphamide or dacarbazine. Owing to pharmacodynamic factors the doses of vincristine, doxorubicine and cisplatinum must be reduced according to the age of the patient. It can be generally stated that the younger the patient the better the tolerance to cytostatic drug treatment.

Die Behandlung von Tumorkrankheiten im Kindesalter ist als Spezialfach innerhalb der Pädiatrie etabliert. Im Gegensatz dazu wurden die besonderen Gesichtspunkte für die Behandlung von Neoplasien des älteren Menschen in Klinik und Forschung bisher kaum untersucht. Entsprechend dürftig ist das Ergebnis einer Bestandsaufnahme auf diesem Gebiet.
Derzeit wird bei älteren Tumorpatienten im Prinzip genauso verfahren wie bei der Behandlung der übrigen erwachsenen Tumorpatienten, nämlich mit Bestrahlung, Operation und/oder Chemotherapie. Die Zumutbarkeit derartiger Maßnahmen ist dem therapeutischen Temperament des jeweiligen Arztes überlassen. Standardisierungen und allgemeine Übereinkünfte, wie beim betagten Tumorpatienten behandelt werden sollte, liegen bisher kaum vor.
Ähnlich wie bei der antimikrobiellen Chemotherapie müssen auch bei der systemischen Tumortherapie die besonderen Gesichtspunkte der therapeutischen Trias: Patient — Tumor-Medikament in ihrem wechselseitigen Bezug berücksichtigt werden. Die pharmakodynamischen und pharmakokinetischen Besonderheiten der Behandlung älterer Tumorpatienten mit den am häufigsten verwendeten Zytostatika soll besprochen werden.
Methotrexat ist ein Folsäure-Antagonist mit einem breiten Anwendungsbereich in der Onkologie, aber auch bei rheumatischer Arthritis und Psoriasis vulgaris. Methotrexat wird vorwiegend renal eliminiert. Bei Hochdosis-Behandlungen (> 1 g) wird ein therapeutisches Drug monitoring gefordert. Bei 122 Hochdosis-Behandlungen wurde nur 1 x eine toxische Reaktion mit ausgeprägten Ulzerationen der Mundschleimhaut beobachtet (Abb. 1). Diese Patientin war 48 Jahre alt, das Alter der übrigen Patienten lag zwischen 16 und 43 Jahren (Mittelwert 22,5 Jahre). Vermutlich hat die altersbedingte Abnahme der renalen Clearance zur Verlängerung der Plasmahalbwertszeit des Methotrexats von 1.5 auf 15 Stunden mit

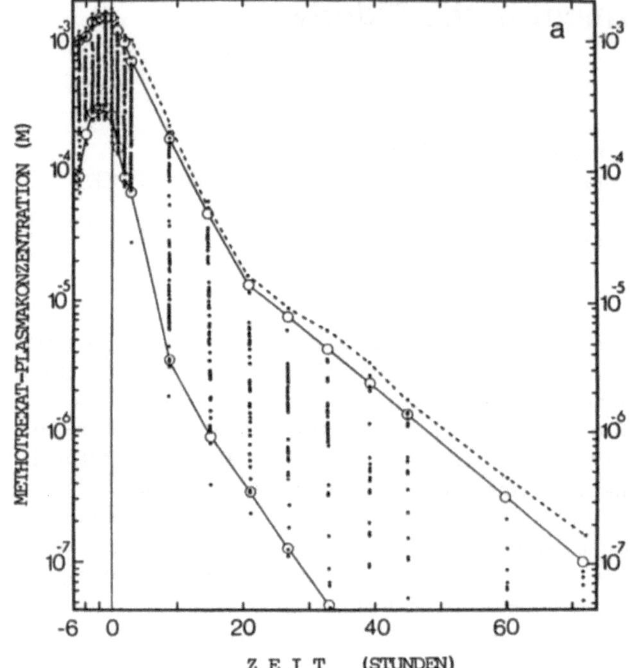

Fig. 1
Scattergramm der Methotrexat-Plasmakonzentrationen bei sieben Patienten mit insgesamt 122 Methotrexatinfusionen von 140 bis 350 mg/kg. Die durchgezogenen Linien geben die 5. und 95. Perzentile der Methotrexat-Konzentrationen wider, die im Verlauf von 121 atoxischen Infusionen gemessen wurden. Die gestrichelte Linie entspricht der einzigen Eliminationskinetik, die eine toxische Reaktion mit schwerer Mukositis nach sich zog (entnommen aus [1]).

beigetragen. Auf Grund einer altersabhängigen Abnahme der renalen Methotrexat-Clearance erhalten Kinder und Jugendliche in den derzeitigen Osteosarkom-Studien 12 g/m^2, Erwachsene lediglich 8 g/m^2 [2, 3].

Der Pyrimidin-Antagonist 5-Fluorouracil wird nur zu 5 % renal und zu über 90 % metabolisch eliminiert. Die totale Clearance beträgt ca. 5 l/min, d.h. die totale Clearance übertrifft um ein Mehrfaches den hepatischen Blutfluß, so daß angenommen wird, daß ein wesentlicher Teil des Metabolismus im extrahepatischen Gewebe erfolgt [4]. Eine verzögerte Elimination bei Leber- oder Niereninsuffizienz ist deshalb nicht beobachtet worden. Besondere Gesichtspunkte bei alten Patienten in Bezug auf Pharmakokinetik und -dynamik sind beim Fluorouracil nicht bekannt.

Die Purin-Antimetabolite 6-Thioguanin, 6-Mercaptopurin und Azathioprin werden sowohl renal als auch hepatisch eliminiert. Dosis-Reduktionen bei Nieren- oder Leberinsuffizienz sollen erforderlich sein [5]. Entsprechende Vorsicht bei älteren Patienten wäre demnach geboten.

Cytarabin, ein Analog zu dem physiologischen Nucleosid Deoxycytidin, ist in seiner phosphorylierten Form ein potenter DNA-Polymerasehemmer. Die Plasmahalbwertszeit des Cytarabin ist kurz (10 min), der größte Teil wird durch eine (hepatische) Deaminase in einen Uracil-Metaboliten (Ara-U) übergeführt. Die Elimination des Ara-U erfolgt weitgehend auf renalem Wege. Während die Elimination von Cytarabin aus Plasma bei 4 Patienten im Alter von 19, 21, 30 und 58 Jahren nahezu deckungsgleich war, konnte bei dem 58-jährigen Patienten eine deutlich verzögerte Elimination des Uracil-Metaboliten nachgewiesen werden (25 Stunden versus 6 Stunden) (Abb. 2 und 3). Da der Uracil-Metabolit

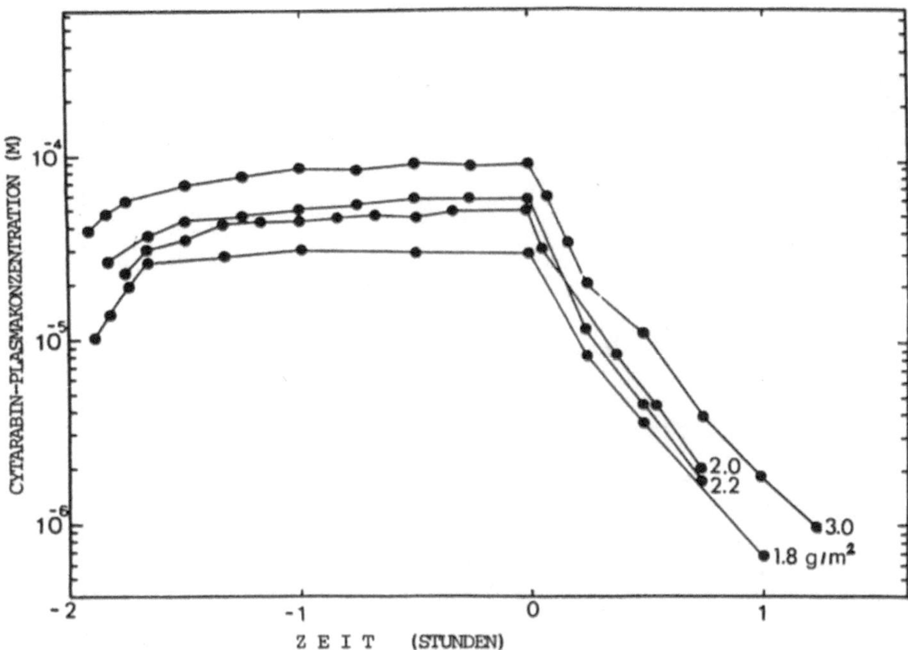

Abb. 2
Zeitlicher Verlauf der Cytarabin-Plasmakonzentrationen während und nach kontinuierlicher zwei-stündiger Cytarabin-Infusionen (1.8 bis 3.0 g/m²) bei vier Patienten im Alter von 19 bis 58 Jahren (entnommen aus [6]).

völlig inaktiv ist, ergibt sich aus seiner verzögerten Ausscheidung keine klinische Konse-quenz. Von pharmakokinetischer Seite sind also bei älteren Patienten keine besonderen Vorsichtsmaßnahmen zu beachten; die erhöhte Knochenmark-Empfindlichkeit limitiert jedoch die Anwendung des Alexans etwas früher als bei jüngeren Patienten.

Von den alkylierenden Zytostatika ist die Phamakokinetik des Cyclophosphamid noch am weitesten untersucht, über die Kinetik der aktiven Metabolite ist jedoch sehr wenig bekannt. Eine Kumulation toxischer Metabolite bei Niereninsuffizienz wurde beobachtet, ohne daß daraus jedoch eine erhöhte toxische Reaktion resultierte [7]. Wir selbst haben die Phamakokinetik des alkylierenden Zytostatikums Dacarbazin (DTIC) bei acht Patien-ten im Alter von 22 bis 57 Jahren untersucht und in Bezug auf die Elimination des DTIC und seines Metaboliten 5-Aminoimidazol-4-carboxamid (AIC) keine Altersunterschiede gefunden [8].

Von den Vinca-Alkaloiden ist in Bezug auf Vincristin die periphere Neurotoxizität der dosislimitierende Faktor. Die Vincristin-Neurotoxizität hängt zwar ab von der kumulati-ven Dosis, sie wird jedoch am häufigsten gesehen bei Patienten über 40 Jahre [9].

Ähnliche Gesichtspunkte gelten für die Kardiotoxizität von Anthrazyklin-Derivaten. Hier gilt neben anderen Faktoren ein Alter über 60 Jahren als fraglicher Risikofaktor. Alters-abhängige Besonderheiten der Pharmakokinetik des Doxo- und Daunorubicins sind bisher nicht bekannt.

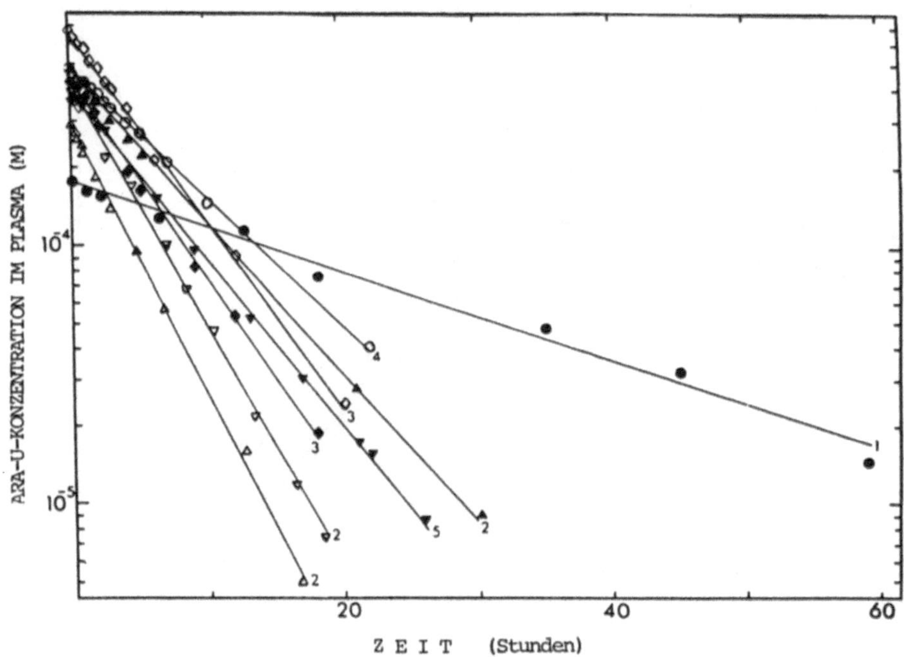

Abb. 3

Zeitlicher Verlauf der Plasmakonzentrationen von 1-β-D-Arabinofuranosyluracil (Ara-U) nach Ende kontinuierlicher zweistündiger Cytarabin-Infusionen (1.8 bis 3.0 g/m²). Bei den Patienten 2 und 3 wurde die Elimination des Uracil-Metaboliten mehrfach untersucht (entnommen aus [6]).

Die Nephrotoxizität des Cisplatinum zwingt bei älteren Patienten von vornherein zur Dosisreduktion. Auch hier sind altersabhängige pharmakokinetische Besonderheiten bisher nicht beschrieben.

Nachdem nun gezeigt wurde, daß die derzeitigen Kenntnisse über pharmakodynamische und pharmakokinetische Besonderheiten der Zytostatika-Behandlung im höheren Alter über das Niveau kasuistischer Mitteilungen noch nicht hinaus sind, soll zum Schluß untersucht werden, inwieweit die verschiedenen Tumoren beim älteren Patienten durch Zytostatika-Behandlungen beeinflußt werden können.

Patienten haben mit zunehmendem Alter eine verminderte Therapietoleranz. Bei akuten myeloischen Leukämien werden bereits bei älteren Kindern niedrigere Remissionsraten und kürzere Überlebenszeiten erzielt als bei Kindern unter 10 Jahren [10]. Die Behandelbarkeit akuter myeloischer Patienten über 65 Jahren wird gerade in einer großen europäischen Studie untersucht. In einer Pilot-Studie mit 240 Patienten mit akuter lymphatischer oder undifferenzierter Leukämie im Alter von 15 bis 65 Jahren hatte sich das Alter als ein prognostisch relevanter Faktor herausgestellt: von den Patienten unter 35 Jahren kamen 49 % in die Vollremission, von den Patienten über 35 Jahre nur 27 % [11]. Bei malignen Non-Hodgkin-Lymphomen mit niedrigem Malignitätsgrad im höheren Alter wird auf Grund der bisherigen Erfahrungen ein abwartendes Verhalten empfohlen, bei hochmalignen Formen ist das zu empfehlende Vorgehen derzeit unklar. Für die Behandelbarkeit des

Morbus Hodgkin stellt das 60. Lebensjahr eine kritische Grenze dar. Bei Plasmozytom-Patienten fanden sich keine Unterschiede im Krankheitsverlauf bei Patienten unter und über 60 Jahren [12].

Zum Schluß noch ein umgekehrtes Beispiel, das zeigen soll, daß bestimmte (hormonell ansprechbare) Tumoren im höheren Alter u. U. auch einmal besser behandelbar sein können: Patientinnen in der Altersgruppe über 50 Jahre profitieren bei der Behandlung des Mamma-Carcinoms im Gegensatz zu prämenopausalen Patientinnen von der Behandlung mit dem Antiöstrogen Tamoxifen [13].

Zusammenfassend läßt sich also sagen, daß bei malignen Systemerkrankungen umso bessere Behandlungsergebnisse erwartet werden können, je jünger die Patienten sind. Die Gründe für die bereits ab den ersten Lebensjahren abnehmende Toleranz gegenüber den Zytostatika sind weitgehend ungeklärt. Neben phamakokinetischen und pharmakodynamischen Gründen werden die im Alter zunehmenden Begleitkrankheiten verantwortlich gemacht.

Literatur

[1] *Breithaupt, H., E. Küenzlen:* Cancer Treat. Rep. 66, 1733–1741 (1982).
[2] *Wang, Y.-M., W. W. Sutow, M. M. Rumsdahl, C. Perez:* Cancer Treat. Rep. 63, 405–410 (1979).
[3] *Rosen, G., R. C. Marcove, B. Caparros:* Cancer 43, 2163–2177 (1979).
[4] *McMillan, W. E., W. H. Wolberg, P. G. Welling:* Cancer Res. 38, 3479–3482 (1978).
[5] *LePage G. A., T. L. Loo:* In: Cancer Medicine, ed. by *J. F. Holland* and *E. Frei* III, p 754, Lea and Febiger, Philadelphia (1973).
[6] *Breithaupt, H., H. Pralle, Th. Eckhardt et al.:* Cancer 50, 1248–1257 (1982).
[7] *Humphrey, R. L., L. K. Kvols:* Am. Assoc. Cancer Res. 15, 84 (1974).
[8] *Breithaupt, H., A. Dammann, K. Aigner:* Cancer Chemother. Pharmacol. 9, 103–109 (1982).
[9] *Praga, C., G. Beretta, L. Vigo et al.* Cancer Treat. Rep. 63, 827–834 (1979).
[10] *Obrecht, J. P.:* In: Hämatologie im Alter, hrsg. von *J. Böhnel, R. Heinz* und *A Stacher*, Seiten 108–113, Urban und Schwarzenberg, Wien (1982).
[11] *Hoelzer, D., E. Thiel, H. Löffler et al.:* Blood 64, 38–47 (1984).
[12] *István, L :* In: Hämatologie im Alter, hrsg. von *J. Böhnel, R. Heinz* und *A. Stacher*, Seiten 167–170, Urban und Schwarzenberg, Wien (1982).
[13] *Fisher, B., C. Redmond, A. Brown et al.:* New Engl. J. Med. 305, 1–6 (1981).

Chronic Diuretic Use in the Elderly

R. Kirsten/B. Heintz/K. Nelson

Department of Clinical Pharmacology, University of Frankfurt, Theodor-Stern-Kai 7, 6000 Frankfurt am Main 70

Summary

The five components of a good hypertensive therapy for the elderly are:
1. Consider therapy if the blood pressure is above 160/90 mm Hg.
2. Try non-pharmacological blood pressure reduction. The two most important are weight reduction and a low salt diet. If these means of reducing blood pressure are unsuccessful, determine renin status.
3. If renin is low, a good response to diuretics can be expected. If renin values are normal or high, a better response to β-blockers may be expected.
4. The diuretic dose should be increased slowly over a period of about 4 weeks until the blood pressure is effectively reduced.
5. Watch for signs of cerebral ischemia and control serum K^+, glucose, uric acid and lipid status every 3 months.

Is Hypertension in the Elderly a Disease?

Some controversy still exists about whether high blood pressure in the elderly is a variant of the norm or a disease [6]. Today the consensus is that hypertension in the elderly is indeed a disease, since it is associated with increased cardiovascular morbidity and mortality [7, 8]. Fig. 1 shows that mortality in the age group from 45 to 54 as well as the age group from 65 to 74 is doubled when the systolic RR is above 160 mm Hg [4]. Fig. 2 shows that men with isolated systolic hypertension in the age group of 75 to 84 are at particularly high stroke risk [3]. The present state of knowledge indicates that treatment of hypertension in the elderly is beneficial in decreasing associated morbidity and mortality [3].

Non-Pharmacological Treatment of Hypertension

The first step in treating hypertension in the elderly is to consider and apply non-pharmacological means, of which the two most important are weight reduction and a low sodium diet. Although the role of a low sodium diet in treating hypertension remains controversial, the beneficial effects appear to be more pronounced in elderly than in younger hypertensives [6, 10]. It has been postulated that high blook pressure may be the result of progressive reduction in renal function, associated with a decreased ability to excrete excess sodium which occurs during the aging process [1], (see Fig. 3). The increase in blood pressure is a compensatory mechanism allowing the impaired kidney to excrete excess sodium. Louwering sodium intake from 150 to 50 mEq/24 hours results in a considerable decrease in systolic blood pressure of about 23 mm Hg in elderly patients with both low and normal renin values, whereas the blood pressure in younger hypertensives remains practically unaffected by this regime [6].

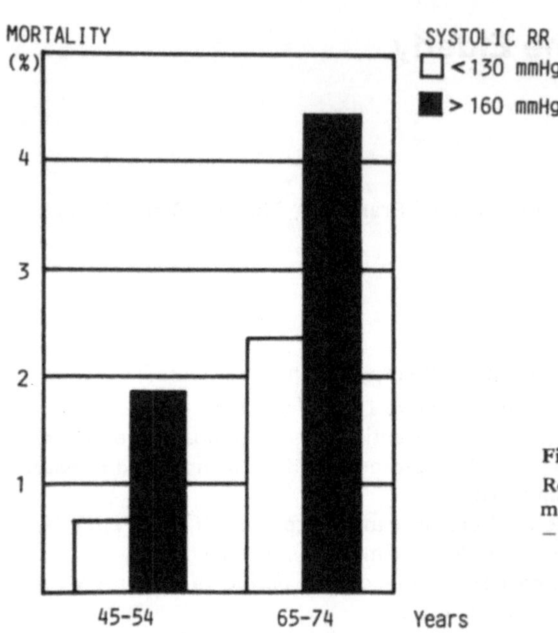

Fig. 1
Relationship of blood pressure to
mortality in two different age groups
— after Kannel and Gordon [4].

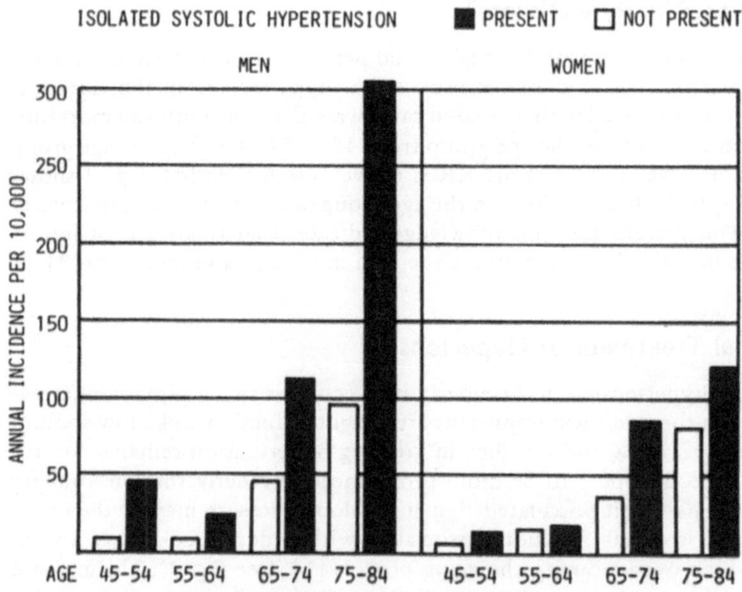

Fig. 2
Relationship of isolated systolic hypertension to stroke risk in men and women in different age groups
— after Kannel [3].

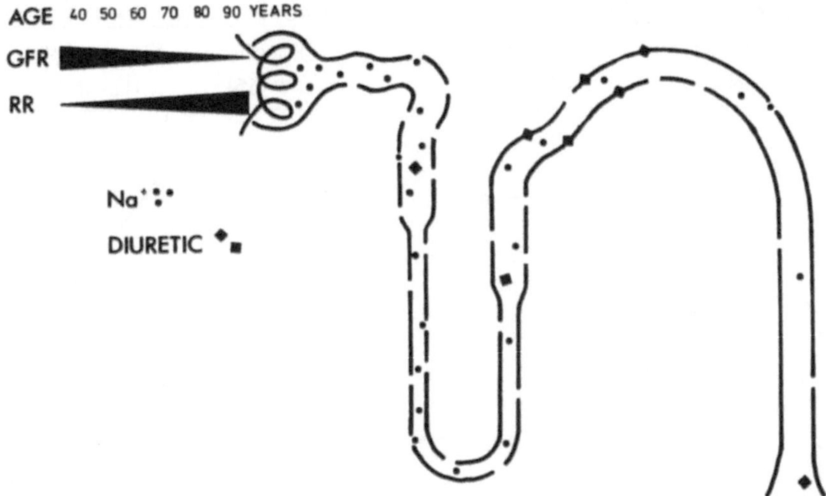

Fig. 3

Inverse relationship of glomerular filtration rate to blood pressure as a function of age. Diuretic blocks Na^+-reabsorption in the tubulus.

Choice of Antihypertensive Drug

If weight reduction or a low sodium diet are not acceptable to the patient or remain ineffective, pharmacological means of blood pressure reduction should be considered. Studies have shown that isolated systolic hypertension in the elderly with low-renin values responds well to diuretics, with an average blood pressure decrease of 31/6 mm Hg [6]. The use of diuretics results in the same effect as reducing sodium intake since re-absorbtion of sodium in the tubulus is inhibited (see Fig. 3). Fig. 4 shows that patients with normal renin values respond better to propranolol than patients with low-renin values who respond better to diuretic treatment. In patients with normal renin values propranolol caused a decrease of 34/7 mm Hg, compared to 22/2 mm Hg induced by diuretics [6].

Minimal Effective Dose

A conservative approach to the elderly hypertensive patient is preferable to complete normalization of blood pressure utilizing potent medication. It is important to remember that hypertension is generally symptomless and that the treatment should also be symptomless. Lack of vascular adaptation coupled with atherosclerotic narrowing of the cerebral arteries in the elderly increases the risk of cerebral ischemia if blood pressure is quickly and drastically reduced. An increase in the occurrence of dizziness, headache, insomnia, confusion, depression or forgetfulness are indications that cerebral ischemia is occurring and should be avoided. The therapeutic goal should therefore be a standing blood pressure of 160/90 mm Hg [3]. The prime object in treating hypertension in the elderly, is to choose a minimally effective dose of a diuretic without producing side effects. Compliance is best when the hypertension can be controlled by a single tablet taken in the morning with breakfast [2].

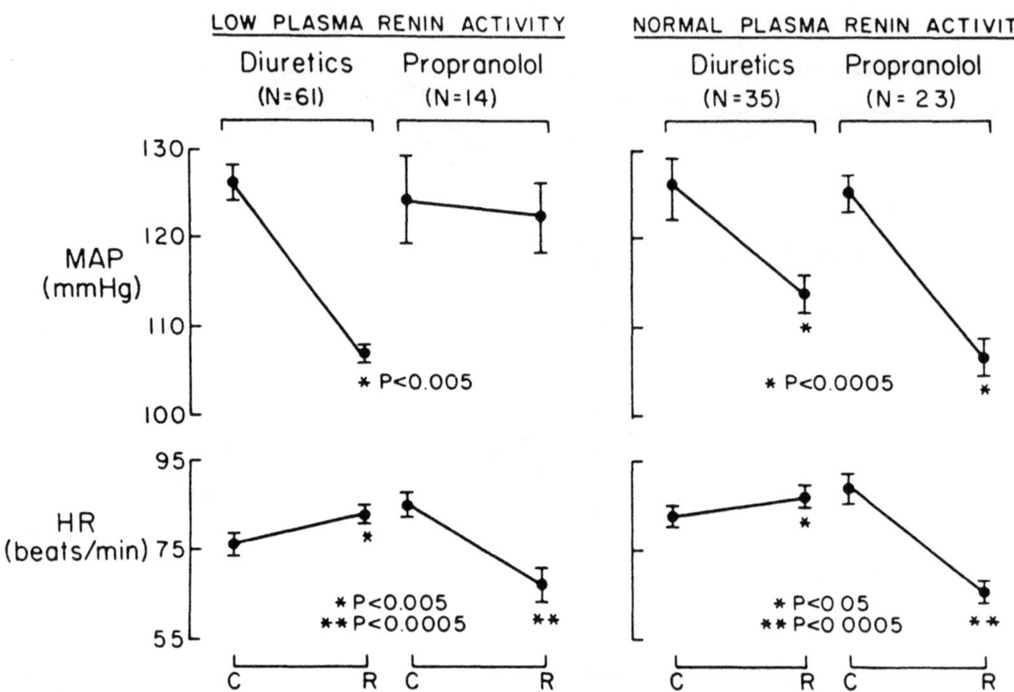

Fig. 4

Comparison of the antihypertensive effect of diuretics and propranolol in low and normal renin essential hypertension of the elderly. MAP = mean arterial pressure; C = control; R = response — after Niarchos [6].

Table I: Problems encountered in diuretic therapy of the elderly — after Messerli [5].

PROBLEMS ENCOUNTERED IN DIURETIC THERAPY	
Pathophysiology in the Elderly:	*Pharmacological Effects of Diuretics:*
Predisposition to sudden ventricular heart death.	Induction of hypokalemia and hypo-magnesia — increased ectopic activity.
Decreased intravascular volume. Impaired baroreceptor function.	Sodium and water deficiency leading to orthostatic hypotension.
Decreased renal blood flow and glomerular filtration rate.	Further decrease in renal blood flow and glomerular filtration rate.
Tendency towards hyperuricemia.	Increase in uric acid.
Tendency towards hyperglycemia.	Increase in glucose intolerance.
Artherosclerosis.	Increase in lipids.

Diuretic treatment in the elderly can be continued for years without adverse side effects. However, it is important to employ the minimal effective dose to ensure that side effects do not occur. Blood pressure, plasma potassium, glucose, uric acid and lipid status should be monitored every three months. After a year of treatment medication may be reduced or stopped. Often blood pressure remains at treatment levels. Should blood pressure increase, reapplication of the diuretic is indicated.

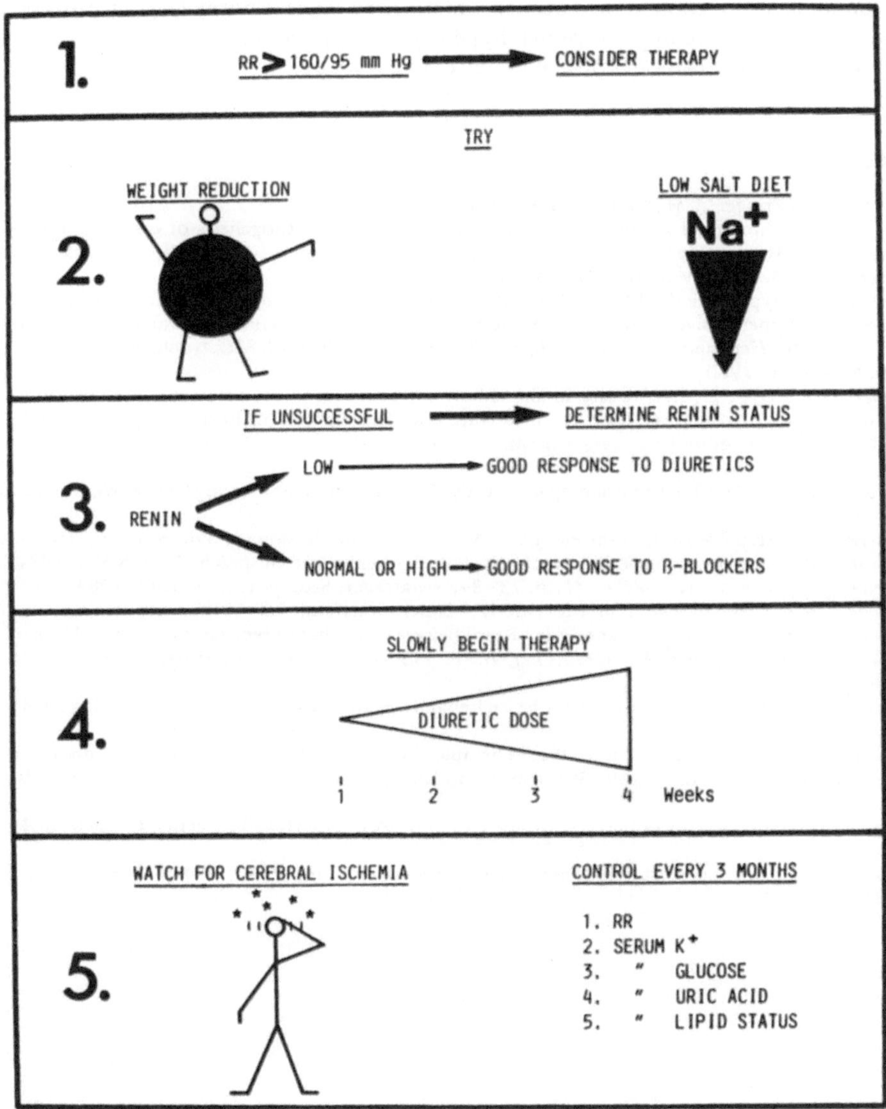

Fig. 5
Five steps in diagnosis and treatment of hypertension in the elderly.

Side Effects

Table I indicates that the problem of diuretic induced side effects in the elderly deserves particular attention since the older organism is more sensitive to particular aspects of some side effects. Hypokalemia may cause increased ectopic activity in patients already predisposed to sudden cardiac arrest. Sodium and water deficiency may lead to orthostatic hypotension which can occur readily in the elderly where a decreased intravascular volume and impaired baroreceptor function occur. Diuretics cause a further decrease in renal blood flow and glomerular filtration rate, both of which occur in the normal aging process. Diuretics tend to exacerbate hyperuricemia, hyperglycemia and atherosclerosis [5].

Fig. 5 lists the five elements of an optimal hypertensive therapy.

References

[1] *Bianchi, G., Caravaggi, A.M., Cusi, D., Barlassina, C., Lupi, G.P., Duzzi, L., Gatti, M., Farrari, P., Velis, O.:* Is an abnormal kidney development involved in the pathogenesis of essential hypertension? In: Hypertension in Children and Adolescents, edited by *Giovanelli, G., New, M., Gorini, S.,* p. 75—88, Raven Press, New York, 1981.

[2] *Hayduk, K.:* Hypertonie-Probleme: Grenzwert- und Altershypertonie, Erfordernishochdruck, Compliance, hypertensiver Notfall. In: Hypertonie — Aktuelle Erkenntnisse Moderne Behandlung, edited by *Heidland, A., Krisch, H.,* p. 27—33, Verlag Gerhard Witzstrock, Baden-Baden, Köln, New York, 1980.

[3] *Kannel, W.B.:* Hypertensive disease in the elderly: A consequence of arteriosclerosis or blood pressure? In: Hypertonie im Alter: Normvariante oder Krankheit?/10. Rothenburger Gespräch, 16—18 Mai, 1984, edited by *Bergener, M., Grobecker, H.,* p. 73—87, Schattauer, Stuttgart, New York, 1984.

[4] *Kannel, W.B., Gordon, T.:* The Framingham Study. U. S. Government Printing Office, Washington D.C., 1974.

[5] *Messerli, F.H.:* Hypertension in the elderly — A defined pathophysiologic Syndrome. In: Hypertonie im Alter: Normvariante oder Krankheit?/10. Rothenburger Gespräch, 16—18 Mai, 1984, edited by *Bergener, M., Grobecker, H.,* p. 73—87, Schattauer, Stuttgart, New York, 1984.

[6] *Niarchos, A.P.:* Hypertension in the elderly: Conclusions and therapeutic implications. In: Hypertonie im Alter: Normvariante oder Krankheit?/10. Rothenburger Gespräch, 16—18 Mai, 1984, edited by *Bergener, M., Grobecker, H.,* p. 179—191, Schattauer, Stuttgart, New York, 1984.

[7] *Ritz, E.:* Auch der Hochdruck im Alter ist zu behandeln. In: Praxis Kurier Selecta-Verlag 18/85 p. 4, 1985.

[8] *Rosenthal, J.:* Stellenwert diuretischer Therapie bei Hochdruck. In: Diuretika, edited by *Rosenthal, J., Knauf, H.,* p. 289—306, edition medizin, Weinheim, Deerfield Beach — Florida, Basel, 1980.

[9] Veterans Administration Cooperative Study Group on Antihypertensive Agents. Circulation 45 (1972), 991.

[10] *Williams, G.:* Salzarme Kost senkt nicht jeden Hypertonus. In: Praxis Kurier Selecta Verlag 36/85, p. 28, 1985.

IV Receptor Changes in the Aged

Pharmakon-Eiweißbindung im Alter: Stopped-Flow Untersuchungen

G. Menke, P. Pfister, S. Sauerwein, B. G. Woodcock
Abt. Klinische Pharmakologie, Klinikum der Universität Frankfurt, Theodor-Stern-Kai 7, 6000 Frankfurt am Main 70

I. Rietbrock
Klinik für Anästhesiologie und Intensivmedizin am Klinikum der Landeshauptstadt, 6200 Wiesbaden

Zusammenfassung

Im Serum von 84 Neugeborenen und Erwachsenen (0–101 Jahre) wurde die Kinetik der Bindung an Humanserumalbumin in Abhängigkeit vom Lebensalter untersucht. Dansylsarkosin (DS) assoziiert spezifisch an der Benzodiazepinbindungsseite von Humanserumalbumin und dient als Modelligand. Die Bestimmung der Bindungskinetik erfolgte in einer Durrum-Gibson Stopped-flow Apparatur über die Aufzeichnung des Zeitverlaufs der Fluoreszenz von Dansylsarkosin während der Bindungsreaktion. Mit einer rechnerischen Anpassung wurden Exponentialfunktionen und Relaxationskonstanten (k_{rel}) aus den Fluoreszenzzeitverläufen ermittelt. Aus diesen konnten die Geschwindigkeitskonstanten für die Assoziation (k_2) und Dissoziation (k_{-2}) sowie die Affinitätskonstanten (K_A, K_A') für die Bindung von Dansylsarkosin an Humanserumalbumin berechnet werden.

Ein signifikanter linearer Zusammenhang besteht zwischen dem Lebensalter und der Assoziationsgeschwindigkeitskonstanten k_2 ($r^2 = 0,59$; $P < 0,001$). Im Serum von Neugeborenen (Mittelwert: $k_2 = 300\ s^{-1}$, $n = 32$) ist k_2 größer als im Serum von Erwachsenen im Alter von 23–65 Jahren ($k_2 = 200\ s^{-1}$; $n = 28$, $P < 0,001$) und von Erwachsenen im Alter von 66–101 Jahren ($k_2 = 144\ s^{-1}$; $n = 24$, $P < 0,001$), so daß die Assoziationsgeschwindigkeit in dieser Reihenfolge abnimmt. Keine wesentliche Altersabhängigkeit besteht für die Geschwindigkeitskonstante k_{-2} ($= 18\ s^{-1}$). Die Affinitätskonstanten K_A sind daher im Alter geringer (Neugeborene: $K_A = 4{,}90 \cdot 10^5$ l/mol; 23–65 Jahre: $4{,}84 \cdot 10^5$ l/mol, n.s.; 66–101 Jahre: $2{,}23 \cdot 10^5$ l/mol, $P < 0,001$).

In Seren mit einem geringen Wert von k_2 wurde eine erhöhte Konzentration an freien Fettsäuren gemessen: es besteht ein deutlicher Zusammenhang zwischen der Abnahme von k_2 und der Zunahme der Konzentration freier Fettsäuren bei alten Menschen. Das molare Konzentrationsverhältnis aus freien Fettsäuren und Humanserumalbumin beträgt im Mittel 0,64 bei Neugeborenen, 0,61 bei Erwachsenen (23–65 Jahre) und 1,40 im Alter (66–101 Jahre, $P < 0,001$).

In einem synthetischen System aus gereinigtem Humanserumalbumin, Dansylsarkosin und Oleat wurde mit fast identischem Ergebnis bestätigt, daß an das Albumin gebundene freie Fettsäuren die Dansylsarkosin-Bindung hemmen. Freie Fettsäuren scheinen somit über einen allosterischen Mechanismus die Konformation an der Benzodiazepinbindungsstelle so zu beeinflussen, daß die Bindungskonstante dort zurückgeht und der ungebundene Anteil des Liganden steigt.

Summary

Human serum albumin is able to specifically bind many endogenous and exogenous substances in blood. The binding kinetics of albumin as a function of age were investigated in serum of 84 subjects (0 to 101 years). Dansylsarcosine (DS) which associates specifically at the benzodiazepine binding site was used as a marker ligand. Binding kinetics were measured in a stopped flow apparatus (Durrum-Gibson) by detection of DS-fluorescence development during the binding reaction. Exponential functions and relaxation constants describing the fluorescence development curves were obtained by curve fitting. Velocity constants for association (k_2) and dissociation (k_{-2}) and binding constants (K_A, K'_A) were calculated.
A significant linear relationship ($r^2 = 0{,}59$, $P < 0.001$) between velocity constant k_2 and age of individuals was obtained. Association is faster in serum of newborn infants (mean: $k_2 = 300\ s^{-1}$, $n = 32$) than in serum from adults (age 23—65 years, $k_2 = 200\ s^{-1}$, $n = 28$, $P < 0.001$) and is slowest in serum of elderly subjects (66—101 years, $k_2 = 144\ s^{-1}$, $n = 24$, $P < 0.001$). The rate of dissociation ($k_{-2} = 18\ s^{-1}$) is not age dependent and so the binding constant K_A decreases with age (newborns: $4.90 \cdot 10^5$ l/mol; 23—65 years: $4.84 \cdot 10^5$ l/mol, ns; 66—101 years: $2.23 \cdot 10^5$ l/mol, $P < 0.001$).
There is a close relationship between k_2 and the concentration of free fatty acids in serum, which increases with age. In newborns and adults (23—65 years) the mean free fatty acid/albumin molar ratios were 0.64 and 0.61 whereas in the elderly the molar ratio was 1.4 ($P < 0.001$).
The role of free fatty acids was confirmed by measurement of the binding kinetics of DS to purified albumin in a synthetic system containing oleate. This showed that free fatty acids apparently have the potential to induce conformational changes at the benzodiazepine binding site of human serum albumin thereby lowering the binding constant and increasing the unbound fraction of drug.

Einleitung

Der Alterungsprozeß des Menschen ist mit physiologischen Veränderungen verbunden, welche die Zusammensetzung des Blutes betreffen (McDonald und McDonald 1982). Obwohl ein Zusammenhang bisher nicht immer aufgeklärt wurde, ist auch die Plasmaeiweißbindung bestimmter Pharmaka beim alten Menschen und beim jungen Erwachsenen unterschiedlich. Die Schwächung der Proteinbindung hat eine Zunahme des ungebundenen Anteils eines Medikaments im Plasmawasser zur Folge. Dies wurde bei älteren Patienten beobachtet für Phenylbutazon (Wallace et al. 1976), für Tolbutamid (Miller et al. 1977), für Warfarin (Hayes et al. 1975) und bei einigen Benzodiazepinen wie Clobazam (Greenblatt et al. 1981), Lorazepam (Divoll und Greenblatt 1982), Temazepam (Divoll et al. 1981) oder Triazolam (Greenblatt et al. 1983). Diese Substanzen werden an den spezifischen Bindungsplätzen des Humanserumalbumins gebunden (Kragh-Hansen 1981), wobei

Warfarin, Tolbutamid und Phenylbutazon an der sogenannten Warfarinbindungsstelle oder Bindungsstelle I assoziieren, die Benzodiazepine an der Benzodiazepinbindungsstelle oder Bindungsstelle II (Sudlow et al. 1976, Fehske et al. 1981, Garten und Wosilait 1972, Müller und Wollert 1973, Brown und Crooks 1976).

Die Kinetik der Bindungsreaktion von niedermolekularen Substanzen und Humanserumalbumin kann mit Hilfe der Stopped-Flow Methode bestimmt werden (Laßmann und Rietbrock 1982, Laßmann et al. 1983). Als Ligand dient Dansylsarkosin, welches mit hoher Spezifität an der Benzodiazepinbindungsstelle assoziiert (Sudlow et al. 1976) und dessen Fluoreszenz sich im Verlauf der Einlagerung in den Komplex verändert. Die Methode ist für Messungen in Nativserum geeignet, da die Gegenwart der übrigen Proteine keinen störenden Einfluß auf die Kinetik der Bindung ausübt (Ulrich et al. 1983). Die Zeitverläufe der Fluoreszenz beim Bindungsprozeß werden aufgezeichnet und ermöglichen nicht nur die Bestimmung der Geschwindigkeit von Assoziation und Dissoziation, sondern auch die Berechnung der Affinitäts- oder Bindungskonstanten für das Bindungsgleichgewicht. Untersucht wurde die Altersabhängigkeit der Bindungskinetik von Dansylsarkosin an Humanserumalbumin in den Seren gesunder Versuchspersonen, um zu klären, ob ein Zusammenhang zwischen der Veränderung physiologischer Parameter im Alter und der Pharmakon-Eiweißbindung für Benzodiazepine im Blut besteht.

Methode

Die Seren wurden aus dem Nabelschnurvenenblut von 32 Neugeborenen und aus dem peripher venösen Blut von 28 Personen aus der Altersgruppe 22—65 Jahre und 24 Personen aus der Altersgruppe 66 bis 101 Jahre gewonnen. Die Blutentnahme bei den Neugeborenen erfolgte direkt nach einer Spontangeburt, bei den Erwachsenen morgens nach zwölfstündiger Nahrungkarenz. Die Bestimmung der klinisch chemischen Blutparameter im Zentrallabor der Universitätsklinik Frankfurt am Main zeigte in keinem Fall eine größere Abweichung vom Normalwert. 6 von 24 Personen der Altersgruppe über 65 Jahre erhielten vor der Blutentnahme Glyceroltrinitrat, Digitoxin, Theophyllin, Glibenclamid oder Doxicyclin, nicht jedoch solche Medikamente mit spezifischer Bindung an der Benzodiazepinbindungsseite des Humanserumalbumins. Die Humanserumalbumin-Konzentration in den Seren wurde mit der Bromkresolgrün-Methode (Rodkey 1965) oder durch Elektrophorese bestimmt, die Konzentration an freien Fettsäuren mit der Methode von Trout et al. (1960) oder Shimizu et al. (1980).

Bestimmung der Bindungskinetik

Die kinetischen Messungen werden in einer Durrum-Gibson Stopped-Flow Apparatur durchgeführt (Laßmann und Rietbrock 1982). Die Vorrats- und Injektionskammern enthalten die beiden Reaktanden Dansylsarkosin und Serum (Abb. 1) in unterschiedlichen Konzentrationsverhältnissen. Nach Auslösen eines Triggerimpulses drückt ein Kolben innerhalb von 2 Millisekunden die Reaktandenlösungen über eine Mischdüse in die Meßzelle. Die zeitliche Änderung der Fluoreszenz wird während der Komplexbildung bei 298 K verfolgt. Die Fluoreszenzanregung erfolgt mit Hilfe einer Xenonhochdrucklampe bei der Wellenlänge 352 ± 3 nm, die Emission wird bei 475 nm gemessen. Die Fluoreszenzzeitverläufe werden mit einem Digitalspeicheroszillographen (Explorer III, Nicolet) aufgezeichnet. Diese Signale werden "on line" auf einen Tischrechner (HP-85, Hewlett-

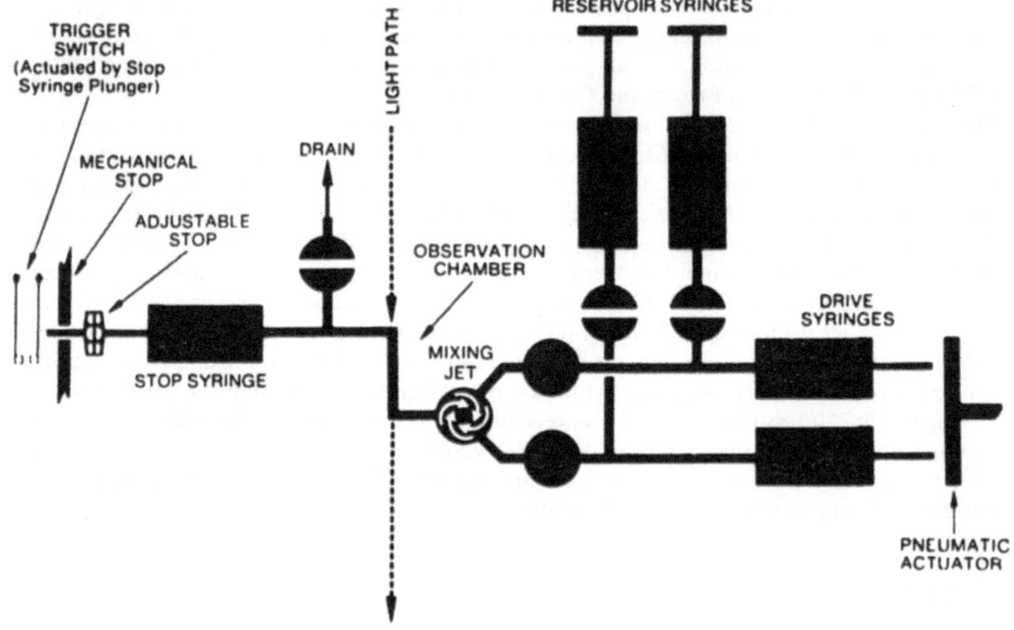

Abb. 1

Aufbau des Stopped-Flow Gerätes (Durrum-Gibson)

Packard) übertragen und mit Hilfe einer "Rotating Iterative Procedure" an zwei vorgegebene Exponentialterme mit den Relaxationskonstanten $k_{obs}1$ und $k_{obs}2$ angepaßt. Da der erste Term zu 90 % und mehr dominiert, geht lediglich $k_{obs}1$ in die weiteren Berechnungen ein.

Reaktionsmodell und Berechnung der Geschwindigkeitskonstanten

Die Reaktion zwischen Dansylsarkosin (DS) und Humanserumalbumin (HSA) verläuft in zwei Teilschritten über ein vorgelagertes Gleichgewicht bis zu einem stabilen Komplex:

$$\text{DS} + \text{HSA} \underset{k_{-1}}{\overset{k_1}{\rightleftharpoons}} \text{DS-HSA}^{\#} \underset{k_{-2}}{\overset{k_2}{\rightleftharpoons}} \text{DS-HSA} \tag{1}$$

k_1, k_{-1}: Geschwindigkeitskonstanten der Hin- und Rückreaktion für Schritt 1
k_2, k_{-2}: Geschwindigkeitskonstanten der Hin- und Rückreaktion für Schritt 2

Im ersten Schritt gelangt Dansylsarkosin durch Diffusion im Plasmawasser an die Oberfläche des Humanserumalbumins und wird dort locker assoziiert (Abb. 2). Die Geschwindigkeit dieses Prozesses ist schnell und ein instabiles vorgelagertes Gleichgewicht ist nach wenigen Millisekunden erreicht. Dieser Teilschritt kann mit der Stopped-Flow Methode nicht verfolgt werden, da er in der Totzeit des Gerätes (2—3 Millisekunden) abgeschlossen ist. Die Umlagerung aus dem instabilen Assoziat DS-HSA$^{\#}$ in einen stabilen Komplex DS-HSA erfolgt wesentlich langsamer. Dieser zweite Schritt ist geschwindigkeitsbestim-

118

mend für die Bindung und nach etwa 100 bis 200 ms abgeschlossen. Aus dem Zeitverlauf der Fluoreszenz nach dem Stillstand der Injektion (Stopped-Flow) bis hin zum Gleichgewichtszustand (Abb. 3) werden die Geschwindigkeitskonstanten k_2 und k_{-2} entnommen. Da kompetitive und/oder allosterische Mechanismen die Geschwindigkeit dieses Schrittes beeinflussen können, erlauben Veränderungen von k_2 und k_{-2} eine Aussage über Hemm- und Aktivierungsmechanismen beim Humanserumalbumin.

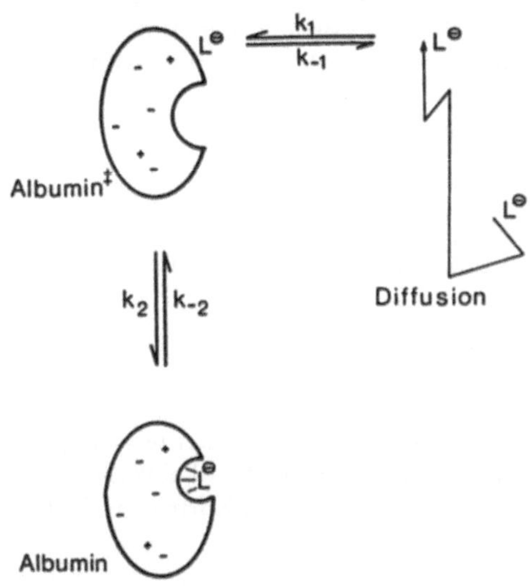

Abb. 2

Reaktionsmodell für die Bindung eines kleinen Liganden (L) am Humanserumalbumin (Albumin) unter Bildung eines spezifischen Komplexes (Albumin-L) mit instabilem Zwischenkomplex Albumin#-L (vergl. Gleichung 1)

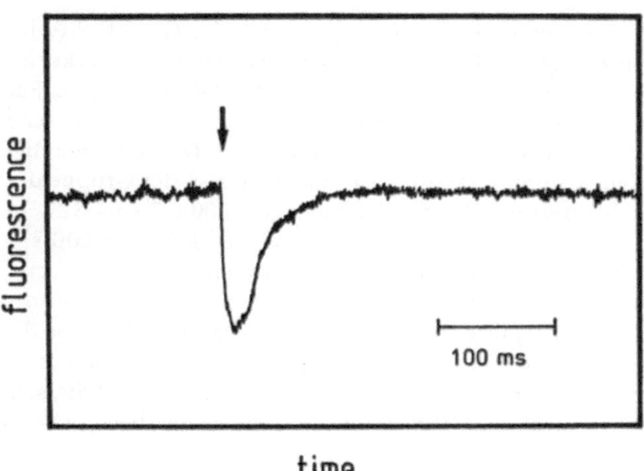

Abb. 3

Bindung von Dansylsarkosin an Humanserumalbumin in Nativserum. Fluoreszenzzeitverlauf (475 nm) bei einem Stopped-Flow Experiment mit $0,055 \cdot 10^{-4}$ mol/l Humanserumalbumin und $0,025 \cdot 10^{-4}$ mol/l Dansylsarkosin in der Meßkammer.
⟶: Injektion der Reaktanden

Unter Berücksichtigung des zugrundegelegten Reaktionsmodelles ergibt sich ein linearer Zusammenhang zwischen der experimentellen Relaxationskonstanten $k_{obs}1$ und den Geschwindigkeitskonstanten k_2 bzw. k_{-2} (Bernasconi 1976):

$$\frac{1}{k_{obs}1 - k_{-2}} = \frac{1}{k_2} + \frac{1}{k_2\, K_A'\, (c_{\overline{DS}} + c_{\overline{HSA}})}. \tag{2}$$

K_A' ist die Affinitäts- oder Bindungskonstante des instabilen Vorkomplexes; $c_{\overline{DS}}$ und $c_{\overline{HSA}}$ sind die Konzentrationen an freiem DS und HSA bei währendem Bindungsgleichgewicht. Aus den Konzentrationsverhältnissen vor der Reaktion und den Relaxationskonstanten $k_{obs}1$ werden die Geschwindigkeitskonstanten k_2, k_{-2} und die Affinitätskonstante K_A' mit der Methode der kleinsten Fehlerquadratsumme angepaßt. Aus diesen angepaßten Werten ergibt sich die Affinitätskonstante K_A:

$$K_A = K_A'\, \frac{k_2}{k_{-2}}. \tag{3}$$

K_A ist die thermodynamische Gleichgewichtskonstante für die Dansylsarkosinbindung an Humanserumalbumin.

Statistik

Bei der statistischen Testung auf signifikante Unterschiede zwischen den Altersgruppen wurden nichtparametrische Verfahren angewendet. Nach einem Kruskal-Wallis-Test folgte die multiple Vergleichsanalyse nach Dunn mit Holm'scher alpha-Korrektur (Dunn 1964, Holm 1979).

Ergebnisse

Die Stopped-Flow Messungen an den Seren von 84 Personen beiderlei Geschlechts im Alter von 0 bis 101 Jahren haben gezeigt, daß die Geschwindigkeit der Dansylsarkosinbindung an Humanserumalbumin signifikant abhängig ist vom Lebensalter (Tab. I). Für die Auswertung wurde das Kollektiv nach den Altersgruppen Neugeborene, Erwachsene des Alters 23–65 und Erwachsene des Alters 66–101 Jahre unterteilt. Die Geschwindigkeit der Umlagerung in den stabilen Komplex DS-HSA ist am größten in der Gruppe der Neugeborenen, die Geschwindigkeitskonstante k_2 beträgt hier etwa $300\ s^{-1}$ (n = 32). In der Altersgruppe 23 bis 65 Jahre ist k_2 signifikant geringer und beträgt etwa $200\ s^{-1}$ (n = 28, P < 0,001) und ist noch geringer in der Gruppe der Personen mit dem Lebensalter 66–101 Jahre, wo ein Mittelwert von $144\ s^{-1}$ (n = 24, P < 0,001) gefunden wurde. Bei 13 von 20 Personen im Alter über 75 Jahre beträgt k_2 weniger als $120\ s^{-1}$. Ohne die Einteilung in Altersklassen kann ein linearer Zusammenhang zwischen k_2 und dem Lebensalter hergestellt werden, der auf dem 0,1 % Niveau signifikant ist ($r^2 = 0,59$, s. u. Abb. 4). In der stetigen Abnahme von k_2 mit zunehmenden Lebensalter besteht kein Unterschied in den Geschlechtern.
Für die Geschwindigkeitskonstante der Dissoziation ist eine zwar signifikante, aber unwesentliche Abhängigkeit vom Lebensalter festzustellen, die Dissoziationsgeschwindigkeitskonstante k_{-2} beträgt für alle Altersklassen etwa $18\ s^{-1}$ (Abb. 4). Das Verhältnis aus den Geschwindigkeiten der Assoziation und der Dissoziation nimmt somit im hohen Alter deutlich ab. Entsprechend geringer sind die Affinitätskonstanten K_A, die im Mittel

Tabelle I: Konzentration von Humanserumalbumin in Serum (c_{HSA}), molares Konzentrationsverhältnis von freien Fettsäuren und HSA (c_{FFA}/c_{HSA}). Geschwindigkeitskonstanten k_2, $k_2 K'_A$ und k_{-2} sowie Affinitätskonstanten K'_A und K_A. Mittelwert (M), Standardabweichung (SD) und Median (Md) für die Altersgruppen Neugeborene, Erwachsene 23–65 Jahre und Erwachsene 66–101 Jahre. Multipler Vergleichstest auf signifikante Unterschiede nach Dunn (Dunn 1964)

		Altersgruppen		
		0 Jahre n = 32	23–65 Jahre n = 28	66–101 Jahre n = 24
c_{HSA} (10^{-4} mol/l)	M SD Md	5,56 0,52 5,45	6,76 0,57 6,90	5,85 0,79 5,95
		——— P < 0,001 ———		
			——— ns ———	
			——— P < 0,001 ———	
c_{FFA}/c_{HSA}	M SD Md	0,64 0,30 0,60	0,61 0,27 0,60	1,40 0,56 1,40
		——— ns ———		
			——— P < 0,001 ———	
			——— P < 0,001 ———	
k_2 (s^{-1})	M SD Md	296 63 300	200 32 196	144 45 145
		——— P < 0,001 ———		
			——— P < 0,001 ———	
			——— P < 0,01 ———	
k_{-2} (s^{-1})	M SD Md	16,3 3,0 16,0	18,4 3,9 18,0	21,0 4,7 18,0
		——— ns ———		
			——— P < 0,001 ———	
			——— ns ———	
$k_2 K'_A$ (10^6 l/mol · s)	M SD Md	7,62 1,78 7,40	8,31 1,92 8,45	4,38 1,64 4,60
		——— ns ———		
			——— P < 0,001 ———	
			——— P < 0,001 ———	
K'_A (10^4 l/mol)	M SD Md	2,69 0,83 2,80	4,24 1,05 4,35	3,19 1,28 3,15
		——— P < 0,001 ———		
			——— ns ———	
			——— P < 0,001 ———	
K_A (10^5 l/mol)	M SD Md	4,90 1,63 4,65	4,84 1,72 5,05	2,23 0,95 2,40
		——— ns ———		
			——— P < 0,001 ———	
			——— P < 0,001 ———	

$4,90 \pm 1,63 \cdot 10^5$ l/mol (M ± SD) für die Neugeborenen, $4,84 \pm 1.72 \cdot 10^5$ l/mol (n. s.) für die Altersgruppe 22—65 Jahre und $2,23 \pm 0,95 \cdot 10^5$ l/mol (P < 0,001) für die Altersgruppe 66—101 Jahre beträgt.

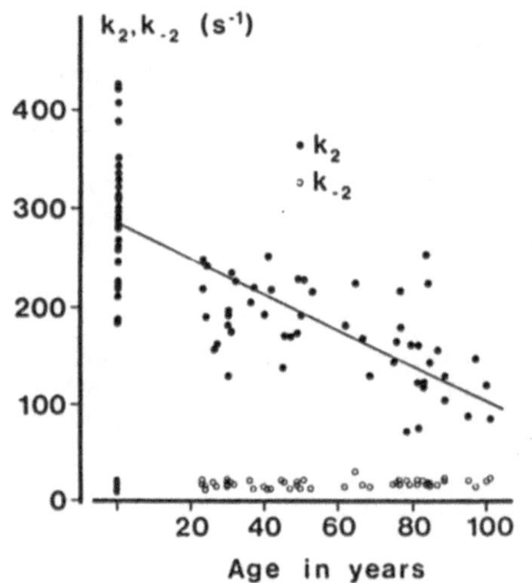

Abb. 4

Geschwindigkeitskonstanten k_2 und k_{-2} für die Bindung von Dansylsarkosin an Humanserumalbumin und Alter bei 84 Versuchspersonen (0—101 Jahre). Lineare Korrelation von k_2 und Alter mit $r^2 = 0,59$ (P < 0,001).

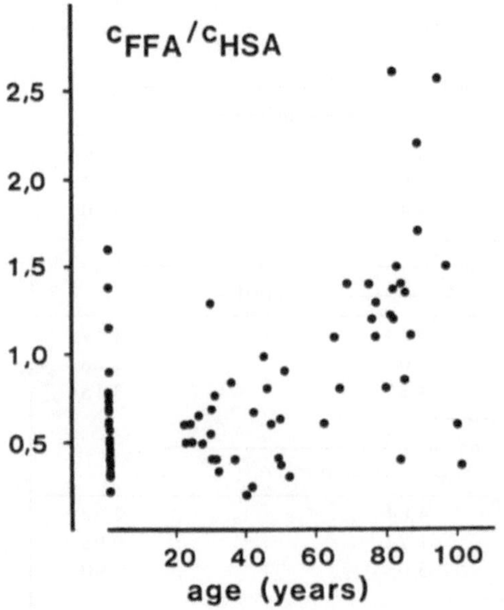

Abb. 5

Molares Konzentrationsverhältnis von freien Fettsäuren und Humanserumalbumin (c_{FFA}/c_{HSA}) und Alter

Die Konzentration des Humanserumalbumins in den Seren ist in den drei Altersgruppen unterschiedlich. Sie ist im Mittel in den Placentarseren (c_{HSA} = 5,56 $\cdot$ 10^{-4} mol/l) und in den Seren der Personen über 65 Jahre (5,85 $\cdot$ 10^{-4} mol/l) geringer als in den Seren der Erwachsenen im Alter von 23–65 Jahren (6,76 $\cdot$ 10^{-4} mol/l, P $<$ 0,001). Für die Konzentration an freien Fettsäuren in den Seren zeigt sich ein eindeutiger Trend zu einer erhöhten Konzentration bei einem Lebensalter über 65 Jahre (Abb. 5). Das molare Verhältnis aus der Fettsäurekonzentration c_{FFA} zur Albuminkonzentration c_{HSA} beträgt bei den Neugeborenen 0,64 und ist damit in etwa gleich groß wie bei den Erwachsenen im Alter unter 65 Jahre. Bei Personen über 65 Jahre ist die Konzentration an freien Fettsäuren im Mittel doppelt so hoch (c_{FFA}/c_{HSA} = 1,4). Bei drei Personen im Alter von 82, 89 und 95 Jahren wurden sogar mehr als 2 mol Fettsäure pro mol Albumin bestimmt.

Diskussion

Der Vergleich zwischen der Geschwindigkeitskonstanten der Umlagerung in den spezifischen Komplex k_2, dem molaren Verhältnis aus Fettsäure- und Albuminkonzentration c_{FFA}/c_{HSA} sowie dem Lebensalter zeigt, daß die reduzierte Geschwindigkeit der Anlagerung des Dansylsarkosins an die Benzodiazepinbindungsstelle mit einer erhöhten Fettsäurekonzentration im höheren Lebensalter einhergeht (Abb. 6). Die Assoziation des Dansylsarkosins schließt offensichtlich Konformationsumwandlungen des Albuminmoleküls ein, die die Geschwindigkeit des zweiten Schrittes (k_2, k_{-2}) mitbestimmen und wesentlich langsamer ist als die diffusionskontrollierte lockere Assoziation. Freie Fettsäuren assoziieren spezifisch an zwei anderen Bindungsstellen des Albumins (Goodman et al. 1958, Spector et al. 1973), welche von der Benzodiazepinbindungsstelle getrennt angeordnet sein sollen (Berde et al. 1979). Die Ligandierung des Albumins an diesen Fettsäurebindungsseiten könnte zu einer veränderten Tertiärstruktur des Albumins führen, aus der die Bildung des Dansylsarkosin-Humanserumalbuminkomplexes erschwert ist und die Geschwindigkeit der Umlagerung (k_2) verlangsamt wird. Der Zusammenhang zwischen k_2

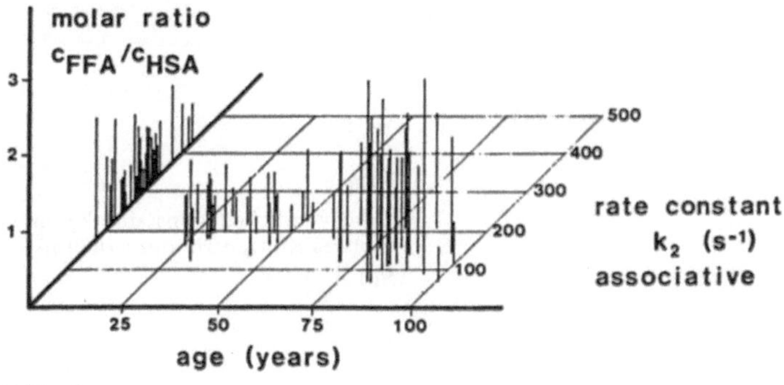

Abb. 6
Geschwindigkeitskonstante k_2, molares Konzentrationsverhältnis c_{FFA}/c_{HSA} und Alter

und dem molaren Verhältnis c_{FFA}/c_{HSA} verdeutlicht (Abb. 7), daß die Besetzung der zwei spezifischen Bindungsstellen für freie Fettsäuren am Albumin eine Verminderung der Geschwindigkeitskonstanten k_2 um den Faktor 4 zur Folge hat. Die Deutung dieser Abhängigkeit als allosterische Hemmung wird unterstützt durch die gute Übereinstimmung mit der Verminderung von k_2, wenn die Ölsäurekonzentration in einem synthetischen System aus isoliertem Humanserumalbumin und Dansylsarkosin schrittweise erhöht wird. Die Variabilität der Einzelwerte bei den Nativseren ist dadurch begründet, daß eine Vielzahl von endogenen und exogenen Substanzen gleichzeitig an HSA spezifisch und unspezifisch gebunden werden (Kragh-Hansen 1981). Jedes dieser Bindungsgleichgewichte kann kompetitiv oder allosterisch die Geschwindigkeit der Dansylsarkosinbindung beeinflussen.

Die Altersabhängigkeit von k_2 stimmt nicht vollständig mit der Altersabhängigkeit der Affinitätskonstanten K_A überein (Abb. 8). Das Reaktionsmodell unterscheidet zwischen der lockeren, eher unspezifischen und der festen, spezifischen Bindung (s. u. Gleichung

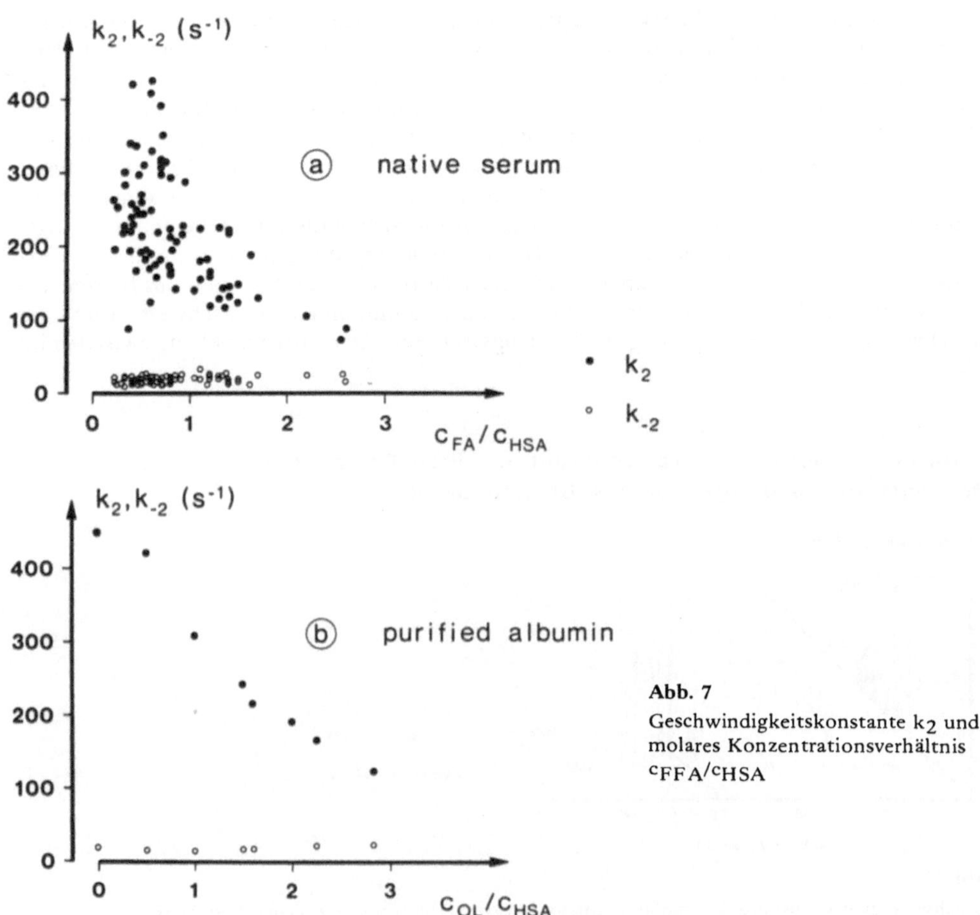

Abb. 7
Geschwindigkeitskonstante k_2 und molares Konzentrationsverhältnis c_{FFA}/c_{HSA}

1—3). Der Unterschied in K_A für die Altersgruppen Neugeborene ($4,90 \cdot 10^5$ l/mol) und
Erwachsene des Alters unter 65 Jahre ($4,84 \cdot 10^5$ l/mol) ist gering, der Unterscheid zwischen den Altersgruppen der Erwachsenen unter und über 65 Jahre dagegen deutlich, die
Bindungskonstante ist bei den über 65-jährigen im Mittel auf etwa die Hälfte reduziert
($2,23 \cdot 10^5$ l/mol, s. u. Tab. I). In Placentarseren tritt vermutlich ein noch nicht bekannter
weiterer Bindungsparameter auf, der die lockere Bindung des Dansylsarkosins an der
Albuminoberfläche kompetitiv stört. Dies kann aus den Bindungskonstanten für das vorgelagerte Gleichgewicht K_A' abgeleitet werden, die bei Placentarseren deutlich geringer
sind als bei Erwachsenen (Tab. I). Die Geschwindigkeit der Bildung des instabilen Vorkomplexes DS-HSA$^{\#}$ ist herabgesetzt, so daß sich im Serum von Neugeborenen die
schnellere Umlagerung (k_2) zum spezifischen Komplex DS-HSA nicht auf K_A auswirken
kann.

Eine Begründung für die deutlich erhöhte Fettsäurekonzentration im Blut alter Menschen
kann noch nicht gegeben werden. Die Eiweißbindung der Benzodiazepine sollte aber bei
Fettsäurespiegeln, die über den Normalwert hinausgehen, geringer sein als bei einem jüngeren Kontrollkollektiv. Die Erhöhung des ungebundenen Anteils einiger Benzodiazepine
in den Seren älterer Patienten wurde bereits bestimmt (Greenblatt et al. 1981, Divoll
und Greenblatt 1982, Divoll et al. 1981, Greenblatt et al. 1983).

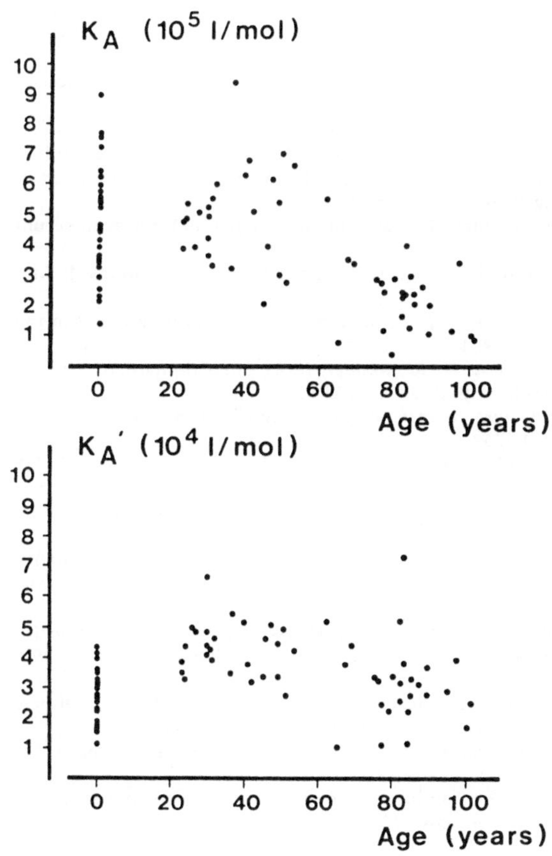

Abb. 8
Affinitätskonstanten K_A' und K_A für
die Bindung von Dansylsarkosin an
Humanserumalbumin und Alter

Der ungebundene Anteil eines Pharmakons im Plasmawasser ist mit seiner Wirkung korreliert. Eine deutliche Verschiebung der Dosis-Wirkungskurve von Benzodiazepinen mit kleinem Verteilungsvolumen und hoher Plasmaeiweißbindung wäre zu erwarten, wenn gleichzeitig mehr als 2 Moleküle an freien Fettsäuren am Albumin gebunden sind. Die kurzfristige Erhöhung des ungebundenen Anteils hat jedoch eine parallele Steigerung der Clearance von Benzodiazepinen zur Folge (Rowland et al. 1983, Rowland 1984). Lediglich bei gleichzeitiger Beeinträchtigung der hepatischen Eliminierung ist eine langanhaltende Zunahme von freiem Benzodiazepin im Blut zu erwarten. Die beim alten Menschen beobachtete niedrigere Albuminkonzentration im Blut (Woodford-Williams et al. 1964) würde diesen Effekt noch verstärken.

Die Unterstützung von Herrn W. Kratzer wird dankbar anerkannt.

Literatur

Berde, C. B., Hudson, B. S., Simoni, R. D., Sklar, L. A.: Human serum albumin. J. Biol. Chem., **254**, 391–400, 1979.
Bernasconi, C. G.: Relaxation Kinetics, Academic Press, New York, 1976.
Brown, K. F., Crooks, M. J.: Displacement of tolbutamide, glibenclamide and chlorpropamide from serum albumin by anionic drugs. Biochem. Pharmacol., **25**, 1175–1178, 1976.
Divoll, M., Greenblatt, D. J.: Effect of age and sex on lorazepam protein binding. J. Pharm. Pharmacol. **34**, 122–124, 1982.
Divoll, M., Greenblatt, D. J., Harmatz, J. S., Shader, R. I.: Effect of age and gender on disposition of temazepam. J. Pharm. Sci., **70**, 1104–1107, 1981.
Dunn, O. J.: Multiple Comparisons using Ranksums. Technometrics, 6, 241–252, 1964.
Febske, K. J., Müller, W. E., Schläfer, U., Wollert, U.: Characterisation of two important drug binding sites on human serum albumin: Rietbrock, N., Woodcock, B. G., Laßmann, A. (eds.) Progress in Drug Protein Binding. Vieweg, Braunschweig/Wiesbaden, p. 5–15.
Garten, S., Wosilait, W. D.: An analysis of the binding of coumarin anticoagulants by human serum albumin. Comp. gen. Pharmacol., 3, 83–88, 1972.
Goodman, D. S.: The interaction of human serum albumin with long chain fatty acid anions. J. Am. Chem. Soc., **80**, 3892–3898, 1958.
Greenblatt, D. J., Divoll, M., Puri, S. K., Ho, I., Zinny, M. A., Shader, R. I.: Clobazam kinetics in the elderly Brit. J. Clin. Pharmacol., **12**, 631–636, 1981.
Greenblatt, D. J., Divoll, M., Abernethy, D. R., Ochs, H. R., Shader, R. I.: Clinical pharmacokinetics of the newer benzodiazepines. Clin. Pharmacokin., **8**, 233–252, 1983.
Hayes, M. J. et al.: Changes in drug metabolism with increasing age: phenytoin clearance and protein binding. Brit. J. Clin. Pharmacol., **2**, 73–79, 1975.
Holm, S.: A simple sequentially rejective multiple test procedure. Scand. J. Statistics., 6, 65–70, 1979.
Kragh-Hansen, U.: Molecular Aspects of ligand binding to serum albumin. Pharmacol. Rev., **33**, 17–53, 1981.
Laßmann, A., Rietbrock, N.: Insight into drug protein binding obtained by stopped-flow measurements. Wyn-Jones, E., Gormally, J. (eds.): Aggregation processes in solution. Studies in physical and theoretical chemistry, **26**, 383–409, 1982.
Laßmann, A., Kratzer, W., Rietbrock, N.: Kinetik der Bindung von Dansylsarkosin (DS) zur Spezifizierung von Humanalbumin (HSA) in Serumkonserven. Fresenius. Z. Anal. Chem., **314**, 487–490, 1983.
McDonald, E. T., McDonald, J. B.: Drug treatment in the elderly. In: Hall, M. R. P. (ed.). Disease Management in the Elderly Vol. 1, Wiley & Sons, Chichester, 1–49, 1982.
Miller, A. K. et al.: Affect of age on the pharmacokinetics of tolbutamide in man. Pharmacologist, **19**, 128, 1977.
Müller, W. E., Wollert, U.: Characterization of the bindung of benzodiazepines to human serum albumin. Naunyn-Schmiedeberg's Arch. Pharmacol., **280**, 229–237, 1973.

Rodkey, F. L.: Clin. Chem., **11**, 478, 1965.

Rowland, M., Leitch, D. S., Fleming, C., Smith, B.: Protein binding and hepatic extraction of diazepam across the rat liver. J. Pharm. Pharmacol., **35**, 383–384, 1983.

Rowland, M.: Protein binding and drug clearance. Clin. Pharmacokin., **9**, 10–17, 1984.

Shimizu, S., Tani, Y., Yamada, H., Tabata, M., Murachi, T.: Anal. Biochem., **107**, 193–198, 1980.

Spector, A. A., Santos, E. C., Ashbrook, J. D., Fletcher, J. E.: Influence of free fatty acid concentration on drug binding to plasma albumin. Ann. NY. Acad. Sci., **226**, 247–258, 1973.

Sudlow, G., Birkett, D. J., Wade, D. N.: Further characterization of specific drug binding sites on human serum albumin. Mol. Pharmacol., **12**, 1052–1061, 1976.

Trout, D. L., Estes, E. H., Friedberg, S. J.: Titration of free fatty acids in plasma: a study of current methods and new modifications. J. Lipid. Res., **1**, 199–202, 1960.

Ulrich, R., Laßmann, A., Kaufmann, R., Rietbrock, N.: Stopped-flow und fluorescenzspektrometrische Untersuchungen des Bindungsverhaltens von Dansylsarkosin an Albumin in Nativserum. Fresenius Z. Anal. Chem., **315**, 534–538, 1983.

Wallace, S., et al.: Factors affecting drug binding in plasma of elderly patients. Brit. J. Pharmacol., **3**, 327–330, 1976.

Woodford-Williams, E., et al.: Serum protein patterns in normal and pathological ageing. Gerontol. Clin., **10**, 86, 1964.

Hypnotics and CNS Function in the Aged Patient

C. G. Swift

Dept. of Health Care of the Elderly, Kings College School of Medicine and Dentistry,
University of London, London, UK

Introduction

Questions concerning the initiation, continuation and cessation of drug treatment have
been widely debated with respect to the managment of insomnia amongst the elderly.
Should drug therapy be used at all? If so, what type of drug and drug regime should be
selected and for how long should treatment be given? This paper will review some of the
available information on the extent and effects of hypnotic use in the elderly and their
relationship to age-related changes in sleep phenomena and in the pharmacokinetics and
pharmacodynamics of hypnotic drugs. Barbiturates and their analogues will not be considered, since it is now recognised that these comparatively unsafe preparations should no
longer be selected for routine use as hypnotics.

Initiation of Treatment

Until fairly recently the rationale for starting hypnotic drugs has received little serious
attention. Patients complaining of insomnia have generally been able to obtain sleeping
tablets from their doctor with few questions asked. Not surprisingly, during the last
decade the scale of prescribing of safe compounds, particularly the benzodiazepines,
achieved massive proportions, the annual rate of increase in the USA at one point being
7 million prescriptions per year [1]. A study of general practice prescribing in the UK
highlighted the frequent prescription of psychotropic drugs in general, but also showed
that the percentage of individuals receiving the three main categories (sedative/hypnotic
drugs, major tranquillisers and antidepressants) rose progressively with advancing age,
reaching a maximum in the over 75's [2]. These figures may to some extent reflect failure
to discontinue treatment rather than numbers of new "cases". However, there is good
evidence that complaints of sleep disturbance are more common in the elderly. A study
of 187 recipients of nitrazepam living in the community [3] identified a range of pre-
cipicating factors leading to the request for a sleeping tablet, most of which could be
classed as problems particularly common in old age (Table I). However, in two-thirds of
patients no "external" cause of sleep disturbance was identified. Several general population surveys have described a number of changes in the pattern of sleep typical of
elderly people, in particular prolonged sleep latency, increased frequency of interrupted
sleep and reduced nocturnal sleep duration [4, 5, 6]. These changes may be partly due to
alterations in life style and basic sleep habits, but there are parallel changes in sleep patterns
recorded on the EEG, in particular loss of the deep, non-REM stages 3 and 4 which
commonly occur early during the night in young individuals [7, 8]. In extreme old age
reduction in REM sleep is also observed [9].

Table I: Factors Precipitating Insomnia and the
Initial requirement for nitrazepam in 187 long-term
recipients [3]

Precipitating Factor	No. of Patients
None	65 (34.8 %)
Bereavement	27
Hospital Admission	20
Pain	18
Own Illness	16
Anxiety, Worry, Fear	12
Other Person's Illness	9
"Environmental"	7
Didn't Know	13

There are thus several contributory factors in the high demand for hypnotic drugs in the elderly, but it is doubtful whether all of these constitute appropriate clinical indications. The associations between both physical and psychiatric illness and sleep disturbance are particularly strong, so that identification of these and their appropriate treatment rather than symptomatic use of hypnotics is particularly important. Alleviation of depressive illness, panic attacks, phobic disorders and organic mental disorders, for example, should be achieved with other forms of therapy, as should the management of psychoses; but all of these conditions may present with insomnia.

The total prescriptions for benzodiazepine drugs in the United Kingdom fell from 19 million to 14 million between 1978 and 1982. This reflected a growing perception that these compounds might not be entirely harmless, in particular that a recognisable state of dependence might occur in some individuals.

Attempts are now being made to define more accurately the clinical indications for hypnotic drugs, which should not be withheld from selected patients who clearly stand to benefit. If underlying causes have been excluded or treated, then careful use of hypnotics is probably appropriate in situations of abnormal stress, as part of an overall regime of controlled psychotropic drug therapy (e.g. in depression) or where short term sleep disturbance poses pratical problems (e.g. to a supporting relative or spouse).

Given an appropriate indication, which drugs should be used and in what dosage? At present, the benzodiazepines and chlormethiazole are probably the only acceptable first line compounds.

Although inter-individual variability in response is high, the elderly are now well known to show increased susceptibility to unwanted sedation if standard adult doses of benzodiazepine hypnotics are administered [10, 11, 12]. This occurs particularly on acute or initial administration before the development of pharmacodynamic tolerance. The fact that this susceptibility can be largely abolished by dose reduction emphasises the importance of pharmacokinetic and pharmacodynamic changes with age in the production of adverse effects (rather than simply the scale of prescribing) with some drugs. With the benzodiazepines, the available evidence points to an increase in pharmacodynamic "sensitivity" of the CNS with age as the major determinant, although alterations in drug handling are also known to occur.

130

Fig. 1a shows the immediate and residual effects of 10 mg of oral diazepam on postural sway in a comparative study of young and elderly healthy volunteers. As expected, base line sway was higher in the old than in the young group, but the sedative effect of diazepam measured in this way was also substantially greater. In spite of the long plasma half life of diazepam, no residual effects were found at this dose, although impairment in performance on the Digit Symbol Subsitution Test in the same study was demonstrable up to 12 hours post dose in the elderly group. The corresponding free (unbound) plasma diazepam concentrations are shown in Fig. 1b. These did not differ between the groups except at 2 and 14 hours, when the level was significantly lower in the elderly subjects. Thus, the accentuated pharmacological effect was not explained by elevated plasma concentrations [13]. Similar evidence from studies of intravenous diazepam for premedication [14, 15, 16] and of oral nitrazepam [17], temazepam [18] and loprazolam [19] has been reported. These findings point to a pharmacodynamic mechanism for the enhanced response. Preliminary data from animal studies indicate no age-related change in benzodiazepine receptor numbers or binding affinity [20]. So far there are no comparable data from human CNS receptor studies, but it seems likely that the mechanism lies distal to the specific receptor site, possibly within other factors affecting chloride channel permeability or some impairment of compensatory mechanisms within the CNS. This argument is supported by the finding of a similar increase in responsiveness to chlormethiazole in the elderly [21].

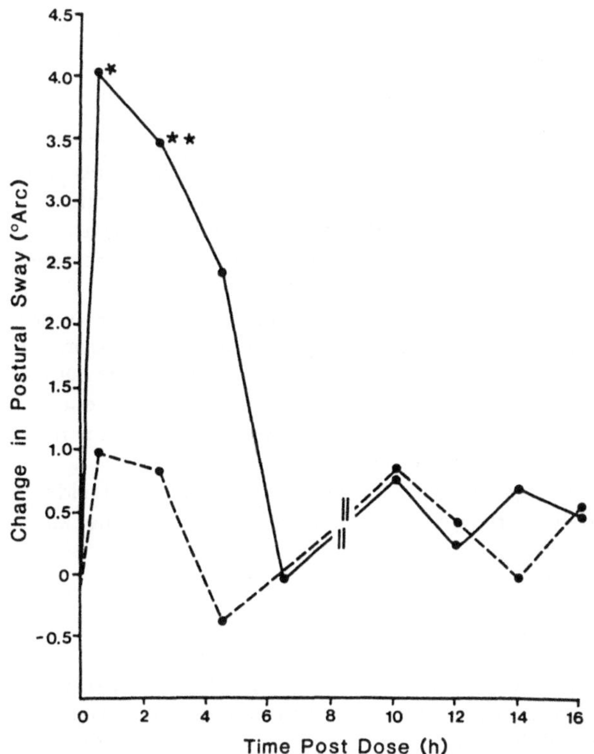

Fig. 1a

Immediate and residual effects of oral diazepam 10 mg on postural sway and

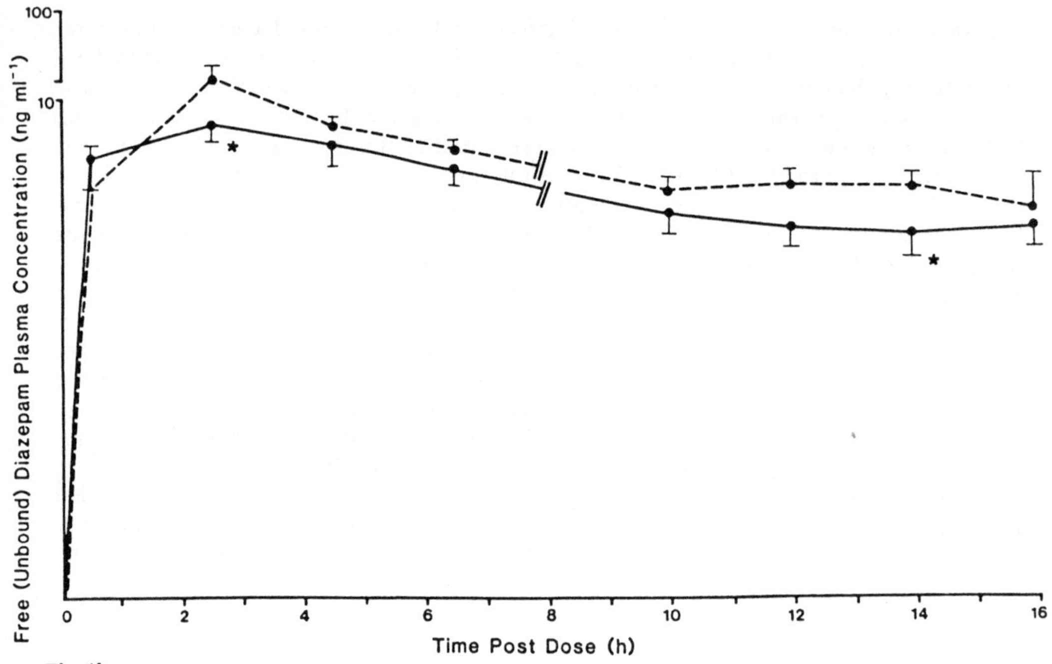

Fig. 1b

corresponding plasma free (unbound) diazepam concentrations, in young (-------) and elderly (—·—) volunteers. (* p < 0.05; ** p < 0.01 between groups). [13]

The plasma half-lives of benzodiazepines eliminated via oxidative metabolic routes tend to be prolonged in the elderly and show significant correlation with antipyrine half-lives [22]. Conversely, benzodiazepines metabolised by other pathways such as conjugation or nitro-reduction show little or no change in pharmacokinetics with age. The increased half-life of the former group is partly due to an increase in apparent volume of distribution. This would be anticipated for such highly lipophilic compounds because of the increase in the ratio of fat to lean body mass in the elderly. Some reduction in clearance has also been found in most cases, particularly in males. In theory one might expect the prolongation of half-life to lead to an increased duration of action. Experimentally, however, this has often not been observed, and in practice, dosage is probably the most important determinant of both response duration and response intensity.

Because of the increased risk of unwanted sedation initiation of treatment of elderly patients with hypnotic drugs should be with not more than 50 % of the normal adult dose.

Continuation of Treatment

There has been a marked tendency in the past for hypnotic drugs, once started, to be taken on a regular nightly basis by patients and subsequently provided on routine prescription by doctors. Habitual taking of sleeping tablets for many years is commonplace.

132

In one community study [3], most individuals had been receiving therapy for between 1 and 11 years. Eighty per cent of these recipients were complying with the explicit or implied instructions on containers to take the tablets every night.

The potential disadvantages of regular, prolonged hypnotic medication include accumulation, tolerance and dependence.

The extent of accumulation depends on the plasma clearance, dose and dose interval with respect to any particular compound. This will be considerable with regular administration of slowly cleared drugs such as nitrazepam, flurazepam (as the active metabolite n-desalkylflurazepam) and diazepam. Distribution volume, however, is not a determinant of the degree of accumulation. As stated above, for a number of lipophilic benzodiazepines, the increase in plasma half-life with age is substantially due to increased distribution volume. Thus, for these compounds, the time taken to reach steady state concentration will be longer, but the level will not be significantly changed. Where there is also a reduction in plasma clearance, the steady state concentration will be correspondingly higher.

Nightly administration of slowly eliminated hypnotics is likely to cause unwanted daytime sedation for a variable period of time from the outset of treatment until the development of pharmacodynamic tolerance. The risk may be reduced by avoiding regular administration, prescribing more rapidly eliminated drugs or reducing dosage.

Patients in the above community study [3] were found to have steady state concentrations of nitrazepam closely predictable from average daily dose. This finding was consistent with the scale of accumulation expected from the repeated nightly use (Fig. 2). In the case of flurazepam recipients, the levels of the active metabolite (n-desalkylflurazepam) were substantially higher than those previously reported in young volunteers, confirming the reduced rate of metabolic clearance (via hydroxylation) of this compound in the elderly.

Tolerance, both pharmacokinetic and pharmacodynamic, was a frequent occurrence in the days of regular barbiturate hypnotic presciption. Gradual attenuation of effect, accompanied by progressive escalation of dosage occurred and was a recognised part of the picture of developing dependence. This syndrome does not occur to the same degree with benzodiazepines, but "tolerance" to unwanted sedation develops fairly quickly.

Assessments of the above long-term nitrazepam and flurazepam recipients for evidence of unwanted sedation showed this to be minimal, in spite of the high steady state plasma concentrations. This was largely based on history taking and clinical examination. However, since falls are a potentially serious consequence of over-sedation in the elderly, postural sway was measured using a Wright(Codoc) ataxiameter. This is known to be a reasonably sensitive measure of drug induced sedation [23]. The extent of postural sway in both nitrazepam and flurazepam groups was within the normal range for age, though the absolute level was significantly higher with flurazepam [3]. These findings suggest the development of side effect "tolerance" after prolonged administration of benzodiazepines and tend to be supported by the experimental findings of other workers [24].

The occurrence of dependence may be inferred from the above findings, but has not been conclusively demonstrated in studies of elderly patients. This would necessitate the demonstration of withdrawal phenomena, in particular rebound insomnia. If anything, the latter has been more commonly observed with regular administration of rapidly eliminated compounds [25]. In the case of ultra-short half-life preparations such as triazolam, rebound withdrawal effects may occur even after a single dose [26]. These problems have been less extensively studied with the non-benzodiazepine compound

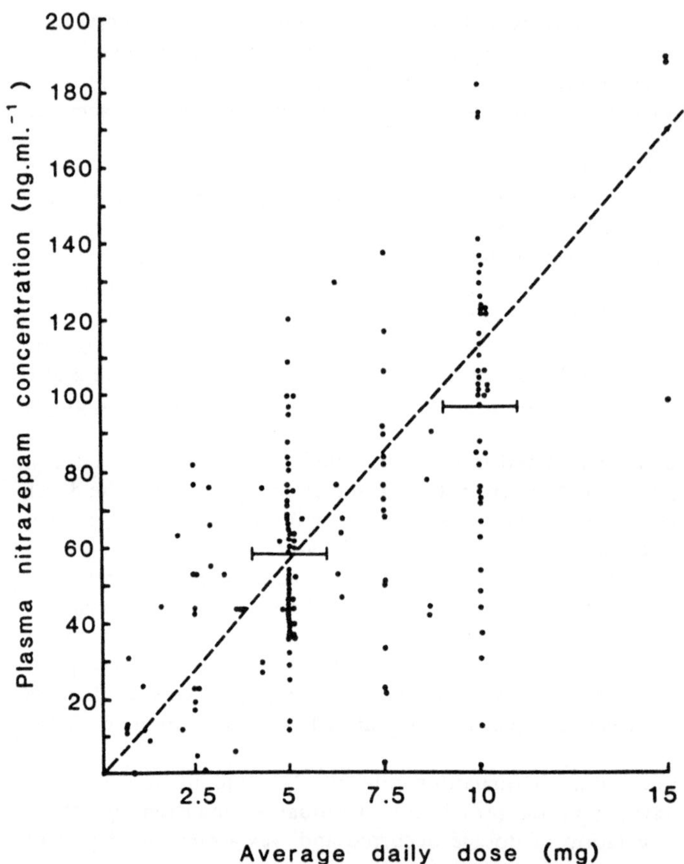

Fig. 2

Plasma "steady state" nitrazepam concentrations in relations to average daily dose in 170 elderly long-term recipients [3].

chlormethiazole (plasma half-life 3—8 hours). Chlormethiazole has a less specific mode of action via GABA-mediated pathways and possibly a direct effect on chloride channel permeability. Reports of significant dependence are largely confined to those with previous or concurrent histories of dependence on alcohol or drugs. Its use as a hypnotic has been predominantly in the elderly over the last two decades. Clinical impressions in this context are that habituation may be less of a problem than with the benzodiazepines. In general it may be concluded that continuation of hypnotic therapy should be neither regular nor prolonged, the emphasis being on short courses and occasional, "if necessary" usage.

Discontinuation of Treatment

The clinical effects of hypnotic therapy should be reviewed within a few days of starting treatment. Careful clinical assessment for any symptoms or signs of unwanted sedation, impaired cognitive function or postural instability should be undertaken. Because of the reduction in homeostatic reserve, such effects in elderly individuals may have serious consequences and their occurrence constitutes an absolute indication to discontinue treatment. Re-introduction of therapy at reduced dosage may subsequently be considered. A substantial proportion of patients will obtain a satisfactory result from the minimum dose, since some degree of placebo response is common.

Only if the drug dosage is completely ineffective and unassociated with adverse effects should an increase in dosage be contemplated. Patients should be counselled about the appropriate use of hypnotics and about their risks. Non-pharmacological alternatives should be considered wherever possible.

No studies have been undertaken of the effects of strategies to withdraw hypnotic therapy in elderly long term recipients, but this has been successfully achieved in isolated cases. While long-term barbiturate consumption may carry specific risks, particularly drug interactions (enzyme induction) and possibly osteomalacia, the comparative safety of the benzodiazepine compounds is perhaps a disincentive to attempts at withdrawal. But the possible adverse sequelae of long term administration (e. g. on cerebral metabolism and function) are unknown and the benefits of such long term use are highly doubtful. The likelihood is that many long term recipients could be successfully withdrawn, given adequate advice and support.

References

[1] Editorial. Benzodiazepines: use, overuse, misuse, abuse? Lancet, (i), 1101. 1973.

[2] *Skegg, D. C. G., Doll, R., Perry, J.:* Use of medicines in general practice. Br. Med. J. 1, 1561–1563, 1977.

[3] *Swift, C. G., Swift, M. R., Hamley, J., Stevenson, I. H., Crooks, J.:* Side effect "tolerance" in elderly long-term recipients of benzodiazepine hypnotics. Age Ageing, 13, 335–343, 1984.

[4] *McGie, A., Russell, S. M.:* The subjective assessment of normal sleep patterns. J. Mental. Sci. 108, 642–654, 1962.

[5] *Karacan, I., Thornby, J. I., Anch, M., Holzer, C. E., Warheit, G. J., Schwab, J. J., Williams, R. L.:* Prevalence of sleep disturbance in a primarily urban Florida county. Soc. Sci. Med. 10, 239–244, 1976.

[6] *Gerard, P., Collins, K. J., Dore, C., Exton-Smith, A. N.:* Subjective characteristics of sleep in the elderly. Age Ageing 7S, 55–59, 1978.

[7] *Feinberg, I.:* Functional implications of changes in sleep physiology with age. In: Terry, R. D., Gershon, S. (ed.) Neurobiology of Ageing. Raven Press, New York, 1976.

[8] *Williams, R. L., Karachan, I., Hursch, C. J.,* In: E. e. g. of human sleep: Clinical Applications. Wiley, New York, 1974.

[9] *Kahn, E., Fisher, C.:* The sleep characteristics of the normal aged male. J. Nerv. Ment. Dis. 148, 477–494, 1969.

[10] Boston Collaborative Drug Surveillance Program: Clinical depression of the CNS due to diazepam and chlordiazepoxide in relation to cigarette smoking and age. N. Engl. J. Med. 288, 277–280, 1973.

[11] *Greenblatt, D. J., Allen, M. D., Shader, R. I.:* Toxicity of high-dose flurazepam in the elderly. Clin. Pharmacol. Ther. 21, 355–361, 1977.

[12] *Greenblatt, D. J., Allen, M. D.:* Toxicity of nitrazepam in the elderly: a report from the Boston Collaborative Drug Surveillance Program. Br. J. Clin. Pharmacol. 5, 407–413, 1978.

[13] *Swift, C. G., Ewen, J. M., Clarke, P., Stevenson, I. H.:* Responsiveness to oral diazepam in the elderly: relationship to total and free plasma concentrations. Br. J. Clin. Pharmacol. 20, 111—118, 1985.

[14] *Reidenberg, M. M., Levy, M., Warner, H., Coutinho, C. B., Schwartz, M. A., Yu, G., Cheripko, J.:* Relationship between diazepam dose, plasma level, age, and central nervous system depression. Clin. Pharmacol. Ther. 23, 371—374, 1978.

[15] *Giles, H. G., MacLeod, S. M., Wright, J. R., Sellers, E. M.:* Influence of age and previous use on diazepam dosage required for endoscopy. Can. Med. Assoc. J. 118, 513—514, 1978.

[16] *Cook, P. J., Flanagan, R., James, I. M.:* Diazepam tolerance effect of age, regular sedation, and alcohol. Br. Med. J. 289, 351—353, 1984.

[17] *Castleden, C. M., George, C. F., Marcer, D., Hallett, C.:* Increased sensitivity to nitrazepam in old age. Br. Med. J. 1, 10—12, 1977.

[18] *Swift, C. G., Haythorne, J. M., Clarke, P., Stevenson, I. H.:* The effect of ageing on measured responses to single doses of oral temazepam. Br. J. Clin. Pharmacol. 11, 413—414P, 1981.

[19] *Swift, C. G., Swift, M. R., Ankier, S. I., Pidgen, A., Robinson, J.:* Single dose pharmacokinetics and pharmacodynamics of oral loprazolam in the elderly. Br. J. Clin. Pharmacol. 20, 119—128, 1985.

[20] *Tsang, C. C., Speed, K. V., Wilkinson, G. R.:* Age and Benzodiazepine binding in the rat cerebral cortex. Life Sci. 30, 343—346, 1982.

[21] *Hockings, N., Stevenson, I. H., Swift, C. G.:* Hypnotic response in the elderly — single dose effects of Chlormethiazole and Dichloralphenazone. Br. J. Clin. Pharmacol. 14, 143P, 1982.

[22] *Greenblatt, D. J., Divoll, M., Abernethy, D. R., Harmatz, J. S., Shader, R. I.:* Antipyrine kinetics in the elderly: prediction of age-related changes in benzodiazepine oxidizing capacity. J. Pharmacol. Exp. Ther. 220, 120—126, 1982.

[23] *Swift, C. G.:* Postural instability as a measure of sedative drug response. Br. J. Clin. Pharmacol. 18, 87S—90S, 1984.

[24] *Campbell, A. J., Somerton, D. T.:* Benzodiazepine drug effect on body sway in elderly subjects. J. Clin. Exper. Gerontol. 4, 341—347, 1982.

[25] *Kales, A., Scharf, M. B., Kales, J. D., Constantin, R., Soldatos, R.:* Rebound insomnia. A potential hazard following withdrawal of certain benzodiazepines. JAMA 24, 1692—1695, 1979.

[26] *Morgan, K., Oswald, I.:* Anxiety caused by a short half-life hypnotic. Br. Med. J. 284, 942, 1982.

Changes in Responses to Drugs Acting on Beta Receptors in Aging

A. J. J. Wood

Departments of Medicine and Pharmacology, Vanderbilt University, School of Medicine, Nashville, Tennessee 37232, USA.

Although the elderly are the principle consumers of therapeutic agents, most of the studies which examine drug efficacy are carried out in young, healthy, usually male, volunteers. Because of both their increasing demographic importance and the frequency with which they receive drugs it is of importance in the future to define the changes which occur in drug response in elderly patients.

One of the systems in which the effects of age have been well studied is the beta adrenergic receptor system. The effects of age on the disposition of the beta adrenergic antagonist propranol has been studied in 27 normal males aged 21—73 years. When unlabelled propranolol was administered orally and ^{3}H propranolol administered simultaneously by the intravenous route it was possible to follow the concentrations in blood samples obtained over the next 8 hours. An effect of age was shown (Fig. 1) in that the mean propranol concentrations in blood were more than two-fold higher in the older group compared to the young [1]. Further examination of the patients revealed that there appeared to be an

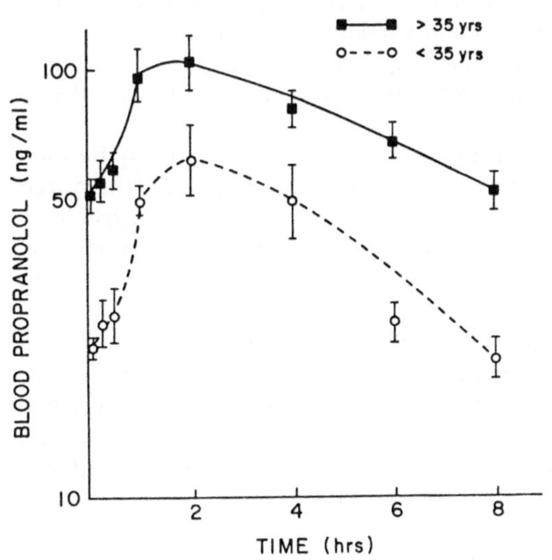

Fig. 1
Steady state blood concentrations of propranolol (mean ± SEM) during 80 mg every & hour administration [1].

Supported in part by USPHS Grants RR95, HL14192, AG01395

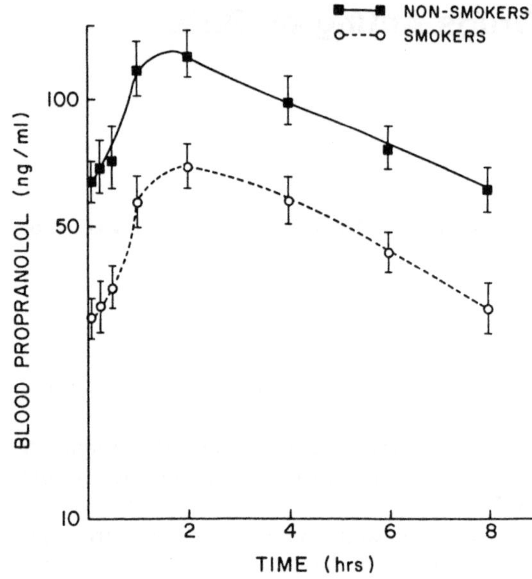

Fig. 2

Propranolol concentrations (mean ±SEM) during oral propranolol (80 mg every & hours) in cigarette smokers and non-smokers [1].

interacting effect of smoking and age on propranolol disposition [1]. Non-smokers had propranolol concentrations which were significantly higher than smokers (Fig. 2). This interaction was reflected in the reduction in the intrinsic clearance of propranolol which occurred with advancing age only in smokers, no such change being seen in non-smokers.

In addition to these dispositional changes seen in the elderly a significant reduction is found in the sensitivity to beta receptor agonists and antagonists in a number of systems [2–8]. Elderly subjects have a smaller chronotropic response to isoproterenol such that the dose of isoproterenol required to raise the heart rate by 25 beats/minute is higher in the elderly than it is in the young [7] (Fig. 3).

This change in beta receptor responiveness seen in aging suggests that there may be some alteration in the beta receptor adenylate cyclase system with advancing age. This system consists of three components: the receptor; the catalytic moiety, which is responsible for catalyzing the synthesis of cyclic AMP, and the guanine nucleotide regulatory unit which communicates the message of hormone binding to the receptor to the catalytic component [9].

It has recently become possible to study beta receptors in humans through the development of assays of radioligand binding to human lymphocyte membranes. The human lymphocyte provides a readily accessible source of tissue which appears to reflect beta receptor activity in other tissues such as the heart [10] and lung. Data has been developed to suggest that the reduced beta adrenergic sensitivity seen in the elderly might be reflected by a reduction in their ability to synthesize adenylate cyclase in response to adrenergic agonists such as isoproterenol [11–13].

Initially it was suggested that this change might be on the basis of alterations in beta receptor density, however, it has since become clear that beta receptor density is unchanged in elderly subjects [14–17].

138

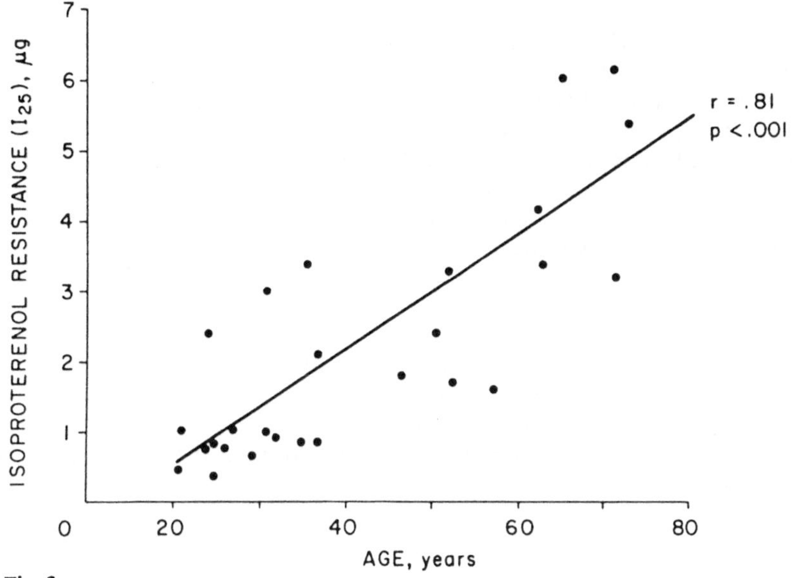

Fig. 3

Relationship between isoproterenol resistance and age [7].

In the face then of an alteration in the adenylate cyclase responsiveness but an absence of change in beta receptor density, it is reasonable to postulate impaired receptor adenylate cyclase communication or beta receptor adenylate cyclase "uncoupling". Uncoupling of the receptor adenylate cyclase complex is seen in the process of receptor densitization and can be quantified by means of radioligand binding techniques using competition binding studies. Densensitization has been shown to be associated with a reduction in receptor affinity for agonists reflecting impaired formation of the high affinity complex of the receptor for agonists [18]. The ability to form the receptor G protein complex is absolutely required for stimulation of adenylate cyclase. Therefore, a reduction in the ability to form this complex will result in reduced adenylate cyclase activity following beta receptor stimulation.

In normal volunteers we have previously shown [19] that receptor adenylate cyclase uncoupling occurs in response to the elevation in catecholamines seen with upright posture in young normal volunteers. Such changes in receptor affinity are in keeping with the previous findings of a rapid change in receptor affinity for agonists in response to increases in catecholamines. Studies subsequently carried out by our group have investigated the role of age and hypertension on receptor adenylate cyclase coupling [17, 20]. Twenty healthy male volunteers aged 21—74 years were studied [17]. All of the subjects had been drug free for at least 10 days and had no abnormality on routine history, physical examination or blood pressure measurement. After overnight supine rest in the hospital an indwelling cannula was inserted and blood samples were drawn for measurement of plasma catecholamines and beta receptor binding of iodohydroxybenzylpindolol. Unlabelled agonist (isoproterenol) was used to compete for the binding of the labeled antagonists and competition binding curves were constructed using 14 different concentrations of isoproterenol. The IC50 of isoproterenol, that is the concentration of isoproterenol which inhibited 50 % of specific antagonist binding, was determined. Examination of the data using computer curve fitting techniques revealed that the receptors in the presence of G.P.P. were a homogeneous population of receptors exhibiting low affinity for agonists. However, in the absence of G.P.P. two populations of receptors could be detected, those exhibiting a high and those exhibiting a low affinity for agonists. Using such computer curve fitting techniques it is possible to determine the proportion of receptors exhibiting the high (% RH) and low (% RL) affinity state for agonists. Age appeared to have a significant effect on agonist binding such that the leukocyte beta receptor affinity for agonists was inversely correlated with age in the 20 subjects (Fig. 4).

This decrease in receptor affinity for agonists with age appeared to be due to a smaller proportion of receptors exhibiting the high affinity state in the elderly subjects than in the young. In the elderly the proportion of receptors binding agonists was high affinity was significantly lower than that seen in young subjects (22.1 % vs. 38.3 % p < 0.05) (Fig. 5). An additional finding was the significant increase in the Kd of the low affinity state with aging while no change occured in the Kd of the high affinity state.

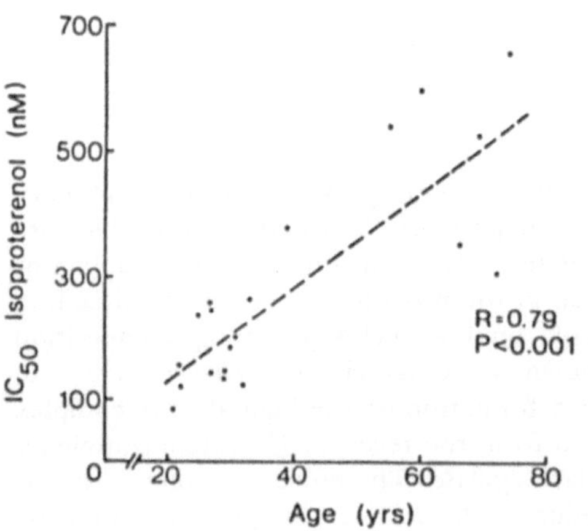

Fig. 4

Correlation between lymphocyte beta receptor affinity for agonists and age. An increase in IC50 represents a reduction in affinity [17].

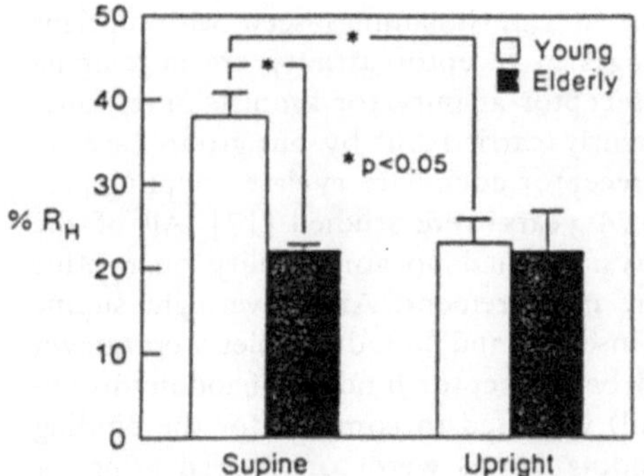

Fig. 5

Effect of posture on the proportion of receptors binding agonists with high affinity (%RH was significantly reduced in the elderly subjects both supine and upright) [17].

Although the explanation for this change is receptor affinity with aging is at this stage unclear, the changes in catecholamines seen with aging may be of some relevance. Plasma norepinephrine and epinephrine were higher in the elderly subjects after overnight supine rest and although they rose by a similar proportion after upright posture, the concentrations in the elderly supine were similar to those seen in the young subjects when they were upright. Thus, one possible explanation for the findings was the elevated plasma catecholamines in the elderly which may have been sufficient to result in receptor desensitization even when the subjects were supine. We, like others, found no change in receptor density with advancing age.

If these changes seen in circulating human lymphocytes are also seen in other more physiologically relevant tissues such as the heart and vasculature, then this might offer an explanation for the reduction in beta receptor function seen in a number of tissues with advancing age.

References

[1] *Vestal, R. E., Wood, A. J. J., Branch, R. A., Shand, D. G., Wilkinson, G. R.:* Effects of age and cigarette smoking on propanolol disposition. Clinical Pharmacology and Therapeutics 26: 8—15, 1979.

[2] *Roth, G. S.:* Changes in hormone binding and responsiveness in target cells and tissues during aging. Adv. Exp. Med. Biol. 61: 195—208 1975,

[3] *Lakatta, E. G.:* Age-related alterations in the cardiovascular response to adrenergic mediated stress. Feld. Proc. 39, 3173—3177, 1980.

[4] *Fleisch, J H., Maling, H. M., Brodie, B. B.:* Beta-receptor activity and cyclic AMP in vascular smooth muscle. Acta. Pharmacol. Toxicol.; 31, Suppl. 1, 45. Abstract, 1972.

[5] *Ericsson, E. E.:* Age dependent variations in β-receptor activity in aorta: variations with age and species. Circ. Res.; 26, 151—162, 1970.

[6] *Lakatta, E. G., Gerstenblith, G., Angell, C. S., Whock, N. W., Weisfeld, M. L.:* Diminished initropic response of the aged myocardium to catecholamines. Circ. Res.; 36, 262—269, 1975.

[7] *Vestal, R. F., Wood, A. J. J., Shand, D. G.:* Reduced β-adrenoceptor sensitivity in the elderly. Clin. Pharmacol. Ther.; 26, 181—186, 1979.

[8] *Bertel, O., Buhler, E. R., Kiowski, W., Lutold, B. E.:* Decreased beta-adrenoreceptor responsiveness as related to age, blood pressure, and plasma catecholamines in patients with essential hypertension. Hypertension; 2, 130—138, 1980.

[9] *Limbird, L. E.:* Activation and attenuation of adenylate cyclase: the role of GTP-binding proteins as macromolecular messengers in receptor-cyclase coupling. Biochem. J.; 195, 1—13, 1981.

[10] *Fraser, J., Nadeau, J., Robertson, D., Wood, A. J. J.:* Regulation of human leukocyte beta receptors by endogenous catecholamines: relationship of leukocyte beta receptor density to the cardiac sensitivity to isoproterenol. J. Clin. Invest.; 67, 1777—1784, 1981.

[11] *Dillon, J., Chung, S., Kelly, J., O'Malley, K.:* Age and beta adrenoreceptor-mediated function. Clin. Pharmacol. Ther.; 27, 769—772, 1980.

[12] *Krall, J. F., Connelly, M., Weisbart, R., Tuck, M. L.:* Age-related elevation of plasma catecholamine concentration and reduced responsiveness of lymphocyte adenylate cyclase. J. Clin. Endocrinol. Metab.; 52, 863—867, 1981.

[13] *Abrass, I. B., Scarpace, R. J.:* Catalytic unit of adenylate cyclase; reduced activity in aged human lymphocytes. J. Clin. Endocrinol. Metab.; 55; 1026—1028, 1982.

[14] *Doyle, V., O'Malley, K., Kelly, J. G.:* Human lymphocyte β-adrenoceptor density in relation to age and hypertension. J. Cardiovasc. Pharmacol. 4, 738—740, 1982.

[15] *Landmann, R., Bittiger, H., Buhler, F. R.:* High affinity beta-2-adrenergic receptors in mononuclear leukocytes: similar density in young and old normal subjects. Life. Sci. 29, 1761—1771, 1981.

[16] *Abrass, I. B., Scarpace, P. J.:* Human lymphocyte beta-adrenergic receptors are unaltered with age. J. Gerontol.; 36, 298—301, 1981.

[17] *Feldman, R. D., Limbird, L. E., Nadeau, J., Robertson, D., Wood, A. J. J.:* Alterations in leukocyte β-receptor affinity with aging. A potential explanation for altered β-adrenergic sensitivity in the elderly. New England Journal of Medicine; **310**, 815–1819, 1984.
[18] *Kent, R. S., De Lean, A., Lefkowitz, R. J.:* A quantative analysis of beta-adrenergic receptor interactions: resolution of high and low affinity states of the receptor by computer modelling of ligand binding data. Mol. Pharmacol.; **17**, 14–23, 1980.
[19] *Feldman, R. D., Limbird, L. E., Nadeau, J., FitzGerald, G. A., Robertson, D., Wood, A. J. J.:* Dynamic regulation of leukocyte beta adrenergic receptor-agonist interactions by physiological changes in circulating catecholamines. J. Clin. Invest.; **72**, 164–170, 1984.
[20] *Feldman, R. D., Limbird, L. E., Nadeau, J., Robertson, D., Wood, A. J. J.:* Leucocyte β-receptor alterations in hypertensive subjects. J. Clin. Invest. **73**, 648–653, 1984.

Pharmakologische Beeinflussung menschlicher β-Adrenozeptoren

O.-E. Brodde

Biochemisches Forschungslabor, Medizinische Klinik & Poliklinik, Abteilung für
Nieren- & Hochdruckkranke, Universitätsklinikum, Hufelandstr. 55,
4300 Essen 1, FRG

Mit Hilfe von Radioligand-Bindungsstudien ist es in den letzten Jahren gelungen, adrenerge Rezeptoren direkt auf molekularer Ebene nachzuweisen [1, 2]. Dabei hat es sich gezeigt, daß die Anzahl adrenerger Rezeptoren (und damit die Ansprechbarkeit des Gewebes auf adrenerge Stimulation) keine starre Größe ist, sondern durch eine Vielzahl von Pharmaka, Hormonen, physiologischen und pathologischen Bedingungen verändert werden kann. Solche Rezeptorveränderungen sind zunächst an einer Reihe von Tiermodellen studiert worden [2], während Studien am Menschen lange Zeit nicht möglich waren, da kein leicht zugängliches, adrenerge Rezeptoren tragendes Gewebe bekannt war. Mit der Entdeckung, daß Lymphozyten β_2-Adrenozeptoren enthalten [3, 4], die excitatorisch an das Adenylat-Zyklase/cAMP-System gekoppelt sind [5, 6] hat sich jedoch die Möglichkeit eröffnet, auch am Menschen Rezeptorveränderungen zu verfolgen. In der vorliegenden Arbeit wurde untersucht, wie physiologische (Alter)- und pharmakologische (Applikation von β-Adrenozeptor-Antagonisten mit und ohne „Intrinsic Sympathomimetic Activity" (ISA) sowie von β-Adrenozeptor-Agonisten)-Einflüsse die Anzahl (bestimmt durch $(-)^{125}$J-Jodocyanopindolol (ICYP) Bindung) und -Ansprechbarkeit (bestimmt als Isoprenalin-vermittelter cAMP-Anstieg) der β_2-Adrenozeptoren in den Lymphozyten gesunder Probanden verändern.

Altersabhängigkeit der lymphozytären β_2-Adrenozeptor-Anzahl und -Ansprechbarkeit

Es ist bekannt, daß im Alter die Ansprechbarkeit mehrerer Rezeptor Systeme auf hormonale Stimulation (Insulin, Glucagon, Prostaglandine, Steroide und Katecholamine) reduziert ist [7]. Um zu untersuchen, ob solche altersabhängige Veränderungen auch für die lymphozytären β_2-Adrenozeptoren gelten, wurde die β_2-Adrenozeptor-Anzahl und -Ansprechbarkeit in den Lymphozyten von 54 jungen männlichen gesunden Probanden (mittleres Alter: 23,5 ± 0,4 (19−30) Jahre), 15 gesunden alten Probanden (10 Männer, 5 Frauen; mittleres Alter: 71,5 ± 2,3 (60−86) Jahre) und 20 Neugeborenen bestimmt [8].

Die mittlere Anzahl der β_2-Adrenozeptoren in den Lymphozyten (bestimmt durch Scatchard-Analyse [9] der ICYP-Bindung) betrug in der Gruppe der jungen Probanden 862 ± 36 (500—1560) spezifische ICYP-Bindungsstellen/Zelle (N = 54); sie war bei den alten Probanden leicht, aber nicht signifikant, höher mit 1230 ± 94 (698—1980) spezifischen ICYP-Bindungsstellen/Zelle (N = 15; Abb. 1). Auf der anderen Seite war die β_2-Adrenozeptordichte in den Lymphozyten der Neugeborenen mit 385 ± 35 (130—608) spezifischen ICYP-Bindungsstellen/Zelle (N = 20) signifikant geringer, während die Affinität des ICYP zu den β_2-Adrenozeptoren für alle drei Altersgruppen nahezu identisch war (Abb. 1).

Der basale cAMP-Gehalt der Lymphozyten war in der Gruppe der jungen Probanden mit 7.0 ± 0.75 pmol cAMP/10^6 Zellen (N = 35) signifikant höher als in der Gruppe der Neugeborenen (5,3 ± 0,55 pmol cAMP/10^6 Zellen, N = 15, P < 0,05; Abb. 2). Der β-Adrenozeptor Agonist Isoprenalin ($10^{-8} - 10^{-4}$ M) führte in allen drei Altersgruppen zu konzentrationsabhängigen Anstiegen des intrazellulären cAMP-Gehaltes, das Maximum des Anstiegs wurde bei 10^{-4} M Isoprenalin erreicht. In den Lymphozyten der Neugeborenen und der alten Probanden jedoch, war der Anstieg des intrazellulären cAMP-Gehaltes bei jeder Isoprenalin-Konzentration signifikant geringer als in der Gruppe der jungen gesunden Probanden (Abb. 2). Während die Affinität des Isoprenalins zu den lymphozytären β_2-Adrenozeptoren (d.h. die Konzentration an Isoprenalin, die nötig ist, um 50 % des maximalen cAMP Anstieges hervorzurufen) bei den jungen Probanden (0.33 ± 0.04 μM) und bei den Neugeborenen (0.22 ± 0.033 μM) nahezu identisch war, war die Affinität des Isoprenalins zu den β_2-Adrenozeptoren bei den alten Probanden (0.94 ± 0.11 μM) signifikant abgeschwächt. Für die Gruppe der Neugeborenen und der jungen Probanden bestand eine signifikant positive Korrelation zwischen der β_2-Adrenozeptor-Anzahl in den Lymphozyten und dem durch 10 μM Isoprenalin hervorgerufenen cAMP-Anstieg (Abb. 3) während für die Gruppe der alten Probanden eine solche Korrelation nicht existierte.

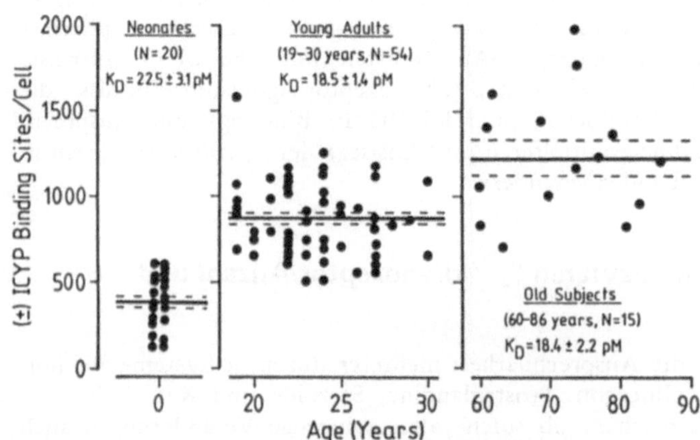

Abb. 1

Anzahl von β_2-Adrenozeptoren — bestimmt durch Scatchard-Analyse [9] der ICYP Bindung — in den Lymphozyten von Neugeborenen (links), jungen (Mitte) und alten gesunden Probanden (rechts).
Ordinate: β_2-Adrenozeptor Anzahl in ICYP Bindungsstellen/Zelle.
Abscisse: Alter (Jahre)
Durchgezogene Linien und gestrichelte Linien: Mittelwerte ± mittlerer Fehler des Mittelwertes des entsprechenden Kollektives. Aus: O'Hara et al. [8]

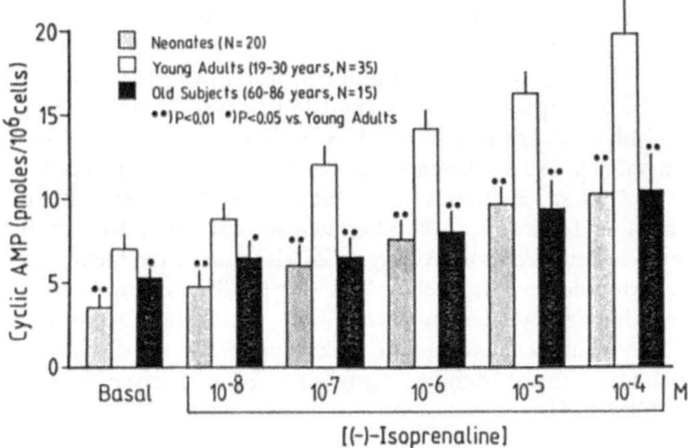

Abb. 2

Einfluß von (−)-Isoprenalin auf den intrazellulären cAMP-Gehalt in Lymphozyten von Neugeborenen (▣), jungen (□) und alten gesunden Probanden (■).
Ordinate: cAMP-Gehalt in den Lymphozyten in pmol cAMP/10^6 Zellen.
Abscisse: molare Konzentration von Isoprenalin
**) P < 0,01, *) P < 0,05 verglichen mit den entsprechenden Werten bei jungen Probanden. Mittelwerte ± mittlerer Fehler des Mittelwertes. Aus: O'Hara et al. [8]

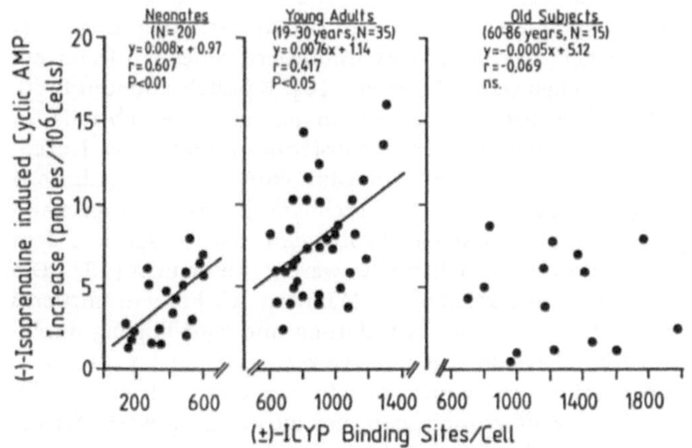

Abb. 3

Korrelation zwischen β_2-Adrenozeptoranzahl und $10 \,\mu$ M (−)-Isoprenalin hervorgerufenem cAMP-Anstieg in Lymphozyten von Neugeborenen (links), jungen (Mitte) und alten gesunden Probanden (rechts).
Ordinate: $10 \,\mu$ M (−)-Isoprenalin hervorgerufener Anstieg des lymphozytären cAMP-Gehaltes in pmol cAMP/10^6 Zellen.
Abscisse: Lymphozytäre β_2-Adrenozeptoranzahl (ICYP Bindungsstellen/Zelle). Aus: O'Hara et al. [8].

Die vorliegenden Befunde zeigen eindeutig, daß mit steigendem Alter die β_2-Adrenozeptordichte in menschlichen Lymphozyten nicht abnimmt, eher leicht zunimmt. Ähnliche Ergebnisse sind auch von anderen Arbeitsgruppen beschrieben worden [10—13]. Die mit steigendem Alter abnehmende β-Adrenozeptoransprechbarkeit [7] ist also nicht auf eine Abnahme der β-Adrenozeptoranzahl zurückzuführen, sondern scheint auf einem „Postrezeptordefekt" zu beruhen. Ein solcher Defekt könnte bei der Kopplung der β-Adrenozeptor-Stimulation zur Adenylat-Zyklase auftreten oder aber die Adenylat-Zyklase selbst betreffen. Abrass und Scarpace [14] konnten kürzlich zeigen, daß beim Menschen die Kopplung von β-Adrenozeptor-Stimulation zur Adenylat-Zyklase im Alter nicht verändert ist, sodaß die im Alter verminderte Ansprechbarkeit der β-Adrenozeptoren auf eine verringerte Aktivierung der Adenylat-Zyklase zurückzuführen ist. In der Tat konnte gezeigt werden, daß Forskolin (eine Substanz, die nicht Rezeptor-vermittelt direkt die Adenylat-Zyklase stimuliert) bei alten Probanden zu signifikant geringeren cAMP-Anstiegen als bei jungen Probanden führt [14].

Einfluß von Terbutalin auf die lymphozytäre β_2-Adrenozeptor-Anzahl und -Ansprechbarkeit

β_2-Adrenozeptor-Agonisten werden häufig in der Therapie obstruktiver Atemwegserkrankungen eingesetzt. Nach langfristiger β_2-mimetischer Behandlung wurde sowohl bei gesunden Probanden als auch bei Asthmatikern ein Abfall der lymphozytären β_2-Adrenozeptordichte beobachtet (Übersicht s. [15]); der resultierende Wirkverlust begrenzt oft die therapeutische Effizienz β-adrenerger Bronchodilatatoren in der Asthmatherapie. Glukokortikoide scheinen bei der Regulation der Dichte und Ansprechbarkeit von β-Adrenozeptoren eine wichtige Rolle zu spielen. So können Glukokortikoide in vivo als auch in vitro die durch β-Agonisten hervorgerufene Desensibilisierung des β-Adrenozeptor/Adenylat-Zyklase Systems abschwächen oder aufheben [16]. Kürzlich konnten Bretz et al. [17] an Ratten zeigen, daß auch Ketotifen, eine antianaphylaktische Substanz, in der Lage ist, eine durch β-Agonisten induzierte Desensibilisierung β-adrenerger Rezeptoren zu verhindern. Wir haben daher den Einfluß von Glukokortikoiden (Prednison) und Ketotifen auf die β_2-Adrenozeptoranzahl und -Ansprechbarkeit (10 μM Isoprenalin hervorgerufener cAMP-Anstieg) in Lymphozyten von Probanden, die 9 Tage mit dem β_2-Agonisten Terbutalin (3 × 5 mg/d oral) vorbehandelt waren, untersucht [18]. Die Studie wurde an 36 gesunden freiwilligen Probanden (26 Männern, 12 Frauen; mittleres Alter: 24.2 ± 0.8 (20—32) Jahre) nach schriftlicher Aufklärung und Einwilligung durchgeführt. Der Versuchsablauf ist in Abb. 4 wiedergegeben: An zwei aufeinander folgenden Tagen vor Beginn der Medikamenteneinnahme wurde den Probanden, nach einer halbstündigen Ruhepause im Sitzen, 30 ml Blut entnommen, um die Ausgangswerte für die lymphozytäre β_2-Adrenozeptordichte und -Ansprechbarkeit zu bestimmen. Danach nahmen alle Probanden für die Dauer von 9 Tagen 3 × 5 mg Terbutalin ein; während dieser Zeit wurden in bestimmten Abständen (gekennzeichnet durch die Pfeile in Abb. 4) Blut entnommen. Nach der letzten Einnahme von Terbutalin wurden die Probanden randomisiert in drei Gruppen eingeteilt: Die erste Gruppe erhielt eine einmalige orale Gabe von 100 mg Prednison, die zweite Gruppe eine Initialdosis von 2 mg und darauf folgend für 4 weitere Tage je 2 × 1 mg/d Ketotifen, während die dritte Gruppe keine weiteren Medikamente erhielt.

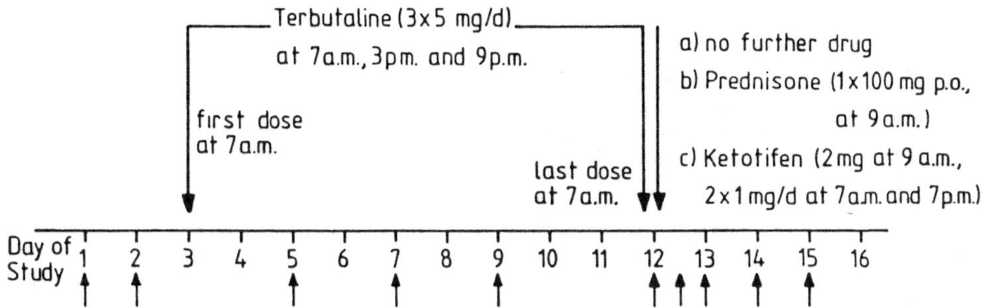

Blood Samples (30 ml heparinized blood for β_2-adrenoceptor number and cyclic AMP response) were taken at 8–10 a.m. after 30 min of rest in sitting position

Heart Rate was measured daily at 8 a.m. and 8 p.m. after 30 min rest in sitting position

Abb. 4
Experimentelles Protokoll der Terbutalin-Studie. Aus: Brodde et al. [18]

Terbutalin führte zu einem raschen Abfall der lymphozytären β_2-Adrenozeptordichte (Abb. 5). Bereits 2 Tage nach Einnahmebeginn des β_2-Agonisten war die Anzahl der β_2-Adrenozeptoren um etwa 40 % abgesunken und blieb während der β-mimetischen Behandlungsdauer auf diesem erniedrigten Niveau. Parallel zur β-Adrenozeptordichte nahm auch der durch 10 μM Isoprenalin hervorgerufene Anstieg des intrazellulären cAMP-Gehaltes in den Lymphozyten ab. Nach Absetzen des Terbutalins nahmen die β_2-Adrenozeptoranzahl und der durch Isoprenalin hervorgerufene cAMP Anstieg nur langsam wieder zu und erreichten erst nach ca. 4 Tagen ihre Ausgangswerte. Eine einmalige orale Gabe von Prednison (100 mg) führte zu einer signifikanten Beschleunigung der Wiederherstellung der Rezeptoranzahl und Ansprechbarkeit: Bereits 8 Stunden nach Einnahme des Glukokortikoids hatten beide Parameter ihre Ausgangswerte wieder erreicht (Abb. 5). Auch Ketotifen (2 mg, danach 2 $\times$ 1 mg) führte zu einer Beschleunigung der Wiederherstellung der β_2-Adrenozeptoranzahl und -Ansprechbarkeit: Bereits 24 Stunden nach der ersten Einnahme von Ketotifen waren beide Parameter auf Werte angestiegen, die nicht mehr signifikant verschieden von den Ausgangswerten waren (Abb. 6). In einer weiteren Versuchsreihe wurde der Einfluß einer gleichzeitigen Gabe von Terbutalin und Ketotifen auf die β_2-Adrenozeptordichte und -Ansprechbarkeit in den Lymphozyten untersucht. Wie Abb. 7 zeigt, verhinderte Ketotifen vollständig die durch Terbutalin hervorgerufene Desensibilisierung der β_2-Adrenozeptoren, die Anzahl der spezifischen ICYP Bindungsstellen/Zelle blieb ebenso konstant wie der Anstieg des cAMP-Gehaltes nach der Stimulation durch 10 μM Isoprenalin. Diese Befunde zeigen, daß Ketotifen und Glukokortikoide in der Lage sind, die Wiederherstellung eines desensibilisierten β-Adrenozeptor/ Adenylat-Zyklase Systems signifikant zu beschleunigen. Darüber hinaus vermag Ketotifen die Desensibilisierung durch β_2-Agonisten zu verhindern. Der genaue Mechanismus dieser beschleunigten Wiederherstellung der desensibilisierten β_2-Adrenozeptoren in den Lymphozyten durch Prednison und Ketotifen ist nicht bekannt. Es ist jedoch in einer Vielzahl von Geweben gezeigt worden, daß eine Langzeitapplikation β-adrenerger Agonisten zu einer Verminderung der Zahl membranständiger Rezeptoren führt (Über-

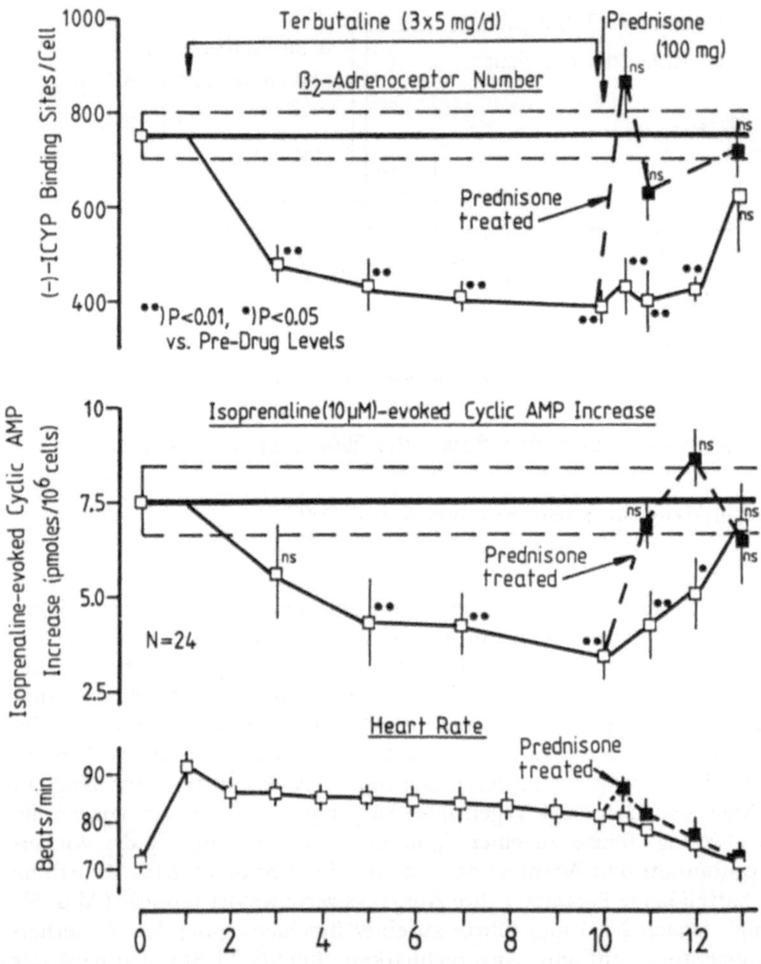

Abb. 5

Einfluß von Terbutalin (3 × 5 mg/d) und Prednison (1 × 100 mg oral) auf β₂-Adrenozeptor Anzahl in Lymphozyten, 10 µM (−)-Isoprenalin hervorgerufenen cAMP-Anstieg in Lamphozyten und Herzfrequenz bei 24 gesunden Probanden.

Ordinate: (von oben nach unten): β₂-Adrenozeptor Anzahl in Lymphozyten — bestimmt durch Scatchard-Analyse [9] der ICYP Bindung — in ICYP Bindungsstellen/Zelle; 10 µM (−)-Isoprenalin hervorgerufener cAMP-Anstieg in Lymphozyten in pmol cAMP/10⁶ Zellen und Herzfrequenz in Schläge/Min. Angegeben sind Mittelwerte ± mittlerer Fehler des Mittelwertes.

Durchgezogene Linien und gestrichelte Linien: Mittelwerte ± mittlerer Fehler des Mittelwertes vor Versuchsbeginn ** P < 0.01 * P < 0.05 verglichen mit den entsprechenden Werten vor Versuchsbeginn. Aus: Brodde et al. [18]

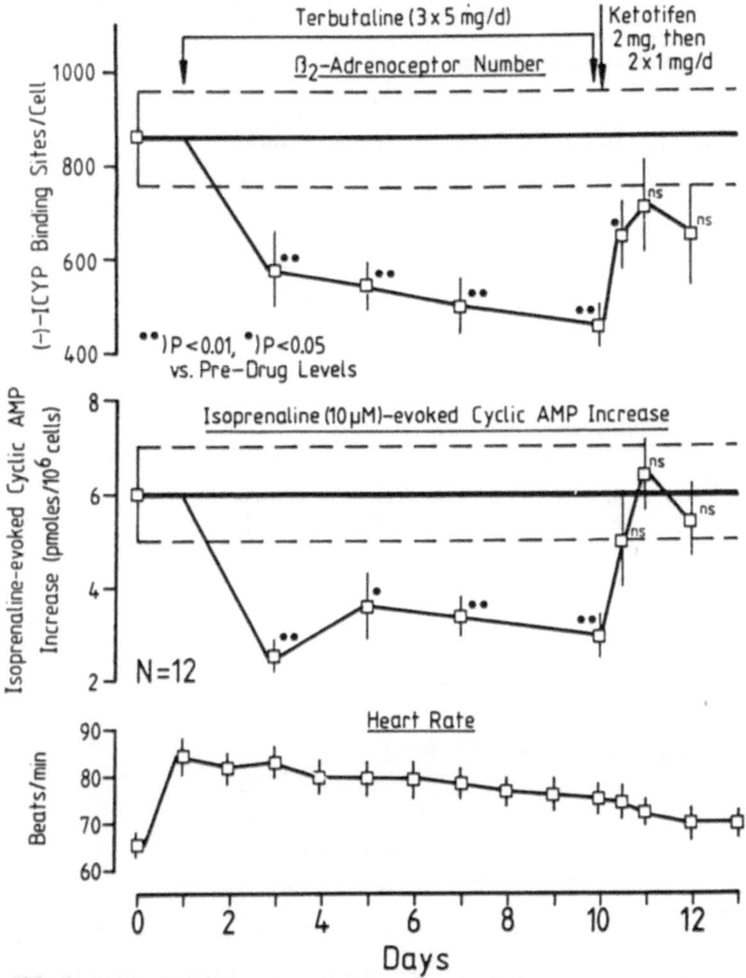

Abb. 6

Einfluß von Terbutalin (3 × 5 mg/d) und Ketotifen (initial 2 mg, danach 2 × 1 mg/d für 4 Tage) auf β_2-Adrenozeptor-Anzahl in Lymphozyten. 10 μM (−)-Isoprenalin-hervorgerufenen cAMP-Anstieg in Lymphozyten und Herzfrequenz bei 12 gesunden Probanden.
Ordinate: (von oben nach unten): β_2-Adrenozeptor-Anzahl in Lymphozyten − bestimmt durch Scatchard-Analyse der ICYP Bindung − in ICYP Bindungsstellen/Zelle; 10 μM (−)-Isoprenalin hervorgerufener cAMP-Anstieg in Lymphozyten in pmol cAMP/10⁶ Zellen und Herzfrequenz in Schläge/Min. Angegeben sind Mittelwerte ± mittlerer Fehler des Mittelwertes. Durchgezogene Linien und gestrichelte Linien: Mittelwerte ± mittlerer Fehler des Mittelwertes vor Versuchsbeginn ** P < 0.01 * P < 0.05 verglichen mit den entsprechenden Werten vor Versuchsbeginn. Aus: Brodde et al. [18].

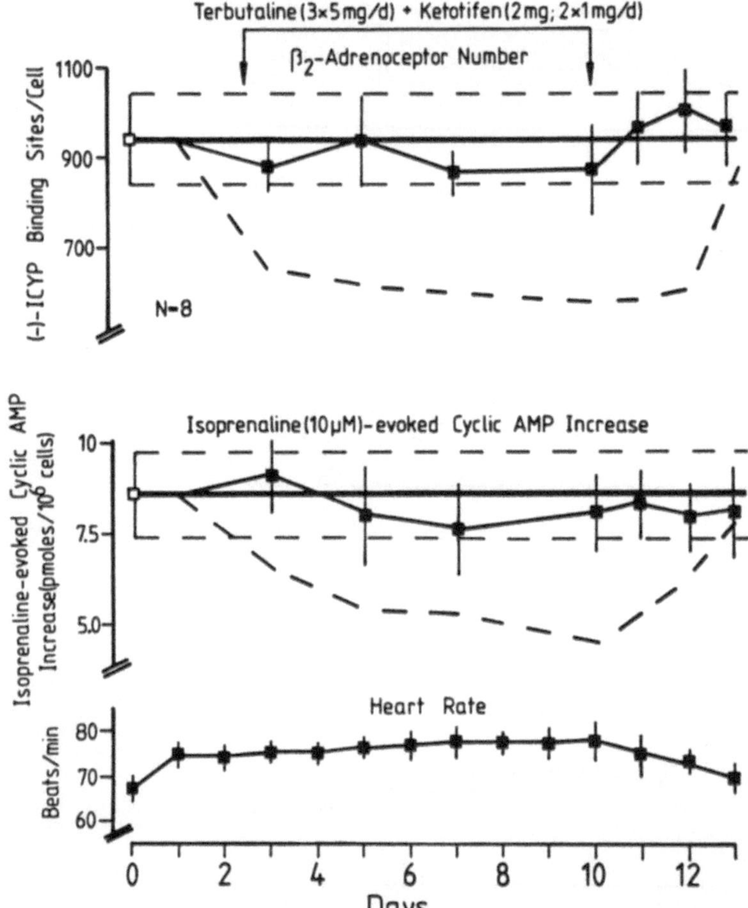

Abb. 7

Einfluß einer gemeinsamen Applikation von Terbutalin (3 × 5 mg/d) und Ketotifen (initial 2 mg, danach 2 × 1 mg/d) auf β_2-Adrenozeptor Anzahl in Lymphozyten, 10 µ M (−)-Isoprenalin hervorgerufenen cAMP-Anstieg in Lymphozyten und Herzfrequenz bei 8 gesunden Probanden.
Ordinate: (von oben nach unten): β_2-Adrenozeptor Anzahl in Lymphozyten − bestimmt durch Scatchard-Analyse [9] der ICYP Bindung − in ICYP Bindungsstellen/Zelle; 10 µ M (−)-Isoprenalin hervorgerufener cAMP-Anstieg in Lymphozyten in pmol cAMP/10⁶ Zellen und Herzfrequenz in Schläge/Min. Angegeben sind Mittelwerte ± mittlerer Fehler des Mittelwertes.
Durchgezogene Linien und gestrichelte Linien: Mittelwerte ± mittlerer Fehler des Mittelwertes vor Versuchsbeginn. Zum Vergleich ist der Effekt von Terbutalin (3 × 5 mg/d) allein (siehe Abb. 5 + 6) in gestrichelten Linien angegeben. Aus: Brodde et al. [18].

sicht s. [15]). Neuere Studien legen die Vermutung nahe, daß im Rahmen dieses Regulationsvorgangs β-Adrenozeptoren „internalisiert" werden, d.h. sie gelangen durch einen endozytotischen Vorgang in das Zellinnere und werden in bislang nicht näher bekannte Zellkompartimente aufgenommen [19]. Es wäre daher denkbar, daß Ketotifen und Glukokortikoide diesen Internalisierungsvorgang hemmen und damit eine Abnahme der lymphozytären β_2-Adrenozeptordichte verhindern.

Die Befunde dieser Untersuchungen über die Regulation β-adrenerger Rezeptoren durch β-Agonisten und deren Beeinflussung durch Prednison und Ketotifen decken sich mit klinischen Erfahrungen aus der Therapie obstruktiver Atemwegserkrankungen. So verlieren adrenerge Bronchodilatatoren bei längerfristigem Einsatz oft an Wirkung, während Glukokortikoide die Ansprechbarkeit auf β-Mimetika wiederherstellen können [16]. Auch an desensibilisierter menschlicher Bronchialmuskulatur konnte eine Wiederherstellung der β-Adrenozeptorfunktion durch Hydrocortison nachgewiesen werden [20]. Da Ketotifen an adrenergen β-Rezeptoren Wirkungen entfaltet, die denen von Prednison sehr ähnlich sind, wird zu prüfen sein, ob z.B. in der Asthmatherapie Glukokortikoide durch Ketotifen ersetzt werden können, wenn β_2-agonistische Bronchodilatatoren nicht mehr die erforderliche therapeutische Wirkung haben. Tatsächlich berichten Lane [21] und Lebeau et al. [22], daß sich nach der Anwendung von Ketotifen die benötigten Glukokortikoiddosen verringerten. Eine entsprechende Dosisreduktion beschrieben auch Kumagai et al. [23] für β-adrenerge Bronchodilatatoren unter Ketotifenzusatz.

Einfluß von β-Blockern auf die lymphozytäre β_2-Adrenozeptor Anzahl

Therapie mit β-Blockern gehört heute zur Basisbehandlung der Hypertonie. Ungeklärt war bisher jedoch, wie sich die sympathomimetische Eigenwirkung (ISA) einiger β-Blocker bei einer solchen antihypertensiven Therapie auswirkt. Um dieser Frage nachzugeben, wurde der Einfluß von Propranolol (nicht-selektiver β-Blocker ohne ISA), Pindolol (nicht-selektiver β-Blocker mit starker ISA) und Bisoprolol (β_1-selektiver Blocker ohne ISA) auf die Anzahl der β-Adrenozeptoren in den Lymphozyten normotensiver Probanden untersucht [24, 25]: 34 gesunde Probanden (30 Männer, 4 Frauen; mittleres Alter: 25.1 ± 2.3 [20–36] Jahre) nahmen an dieser Studie teil. Der Versuchsablauf war wie folgt: An zwei Tagen vor der β-Blocker Einnahme wurde den Probanden 20 ml Heparin-Blut für die β_2-Adrenozeptorbestimmung in den Lymphozyten und 10 ml eiskaltes EDTA Blut zur Bestimmung der Plasma-Renin-Aktivität (PRA) entnommen. Am dritten Tage wurde mit der β-Blocker Einnahme (Propranolol 4×40 mg/Tag; Pindolol 2×5 mg/Tag; Bisoprolol 1×10 mg/Tag) begonnen. Die Einnahmezeiten waren: für Propranolol 6, 12, 18 und 24 Uhr, für Pindolol 7 und 19 Uhr und für Bisoprolol 19 Uhr. Während der Behandlung und nach Absetzen der β-Blocker wurde zu bestimmten Zeitpunkten 20 ml Heparin Blut und 10 ml EDTA-Blut entnommen. Die Blutentnahme erfolgte immer morgens zwischen 8 und 9 Uhr, nach einer halben Stunde Ruhe im Sitzen. Während des gesamten Versuchsablaufs wurden Blutdruck und Herzfrequenz von den Probanden selbst gemessen.

Propranolol (4×40 mg/Tag für 9 Tage) führte bei den Probanden zu einem signifikanten Anstieg der β_2-Adrenozeptordichte in den Lymphozyten, der nach 2 Tagen ca. $30–35\,\%$ betrug (Abb. 8). Ähnliche Effekte von Propranolol auf die β_2-Adrenozeptordichte in den Lymphozyten gesunder Probanden sind auch von Aarons et al. [26] und Wood et al. [27]

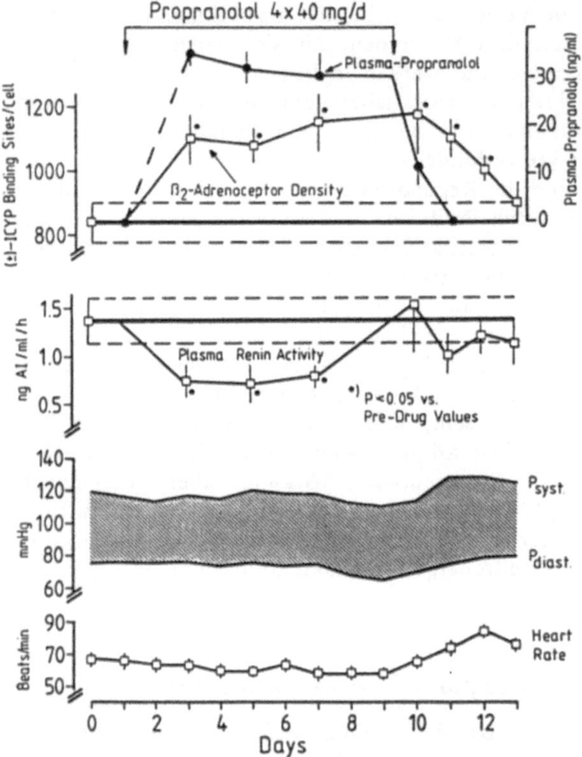

Abb. 8

Einfluß von Propranolol (4 × 40 mg/d) auf β_2-Adrenozeptor-Anzahl, Plasma-Renin-Aktivität, Blutdruck und Herzfrequenz bei 6 gesunden Probanden.

Ordinate: (von oben nach unten): β_2-Adrenozeptor-Anzahl in Lymphozyten — bestimmt durch Scatchard-Analyse [9] der ICYP Bindung — in ICYP Bindungsstellen/Zelle; Plasma-Renin-Aktivität in ng Angiotensin I gebildet/ml/Stunde; Blutdruck in mmHg und Herzfrequenz in Schläge/Min. *rechts:* Plasma-Propranolol-Spiegel in ng/ml.

Abscisse: Versuchstage

Angegeben sind Mittelwerte ± mittlerer Fehler des Mittelwertes.

Durchgezogene Linien und gestrichelte Linien: Mittelwerte ± mittlerer Fehler des Mittelwertes vor Propranolol-Einnahme. *) P < 0.05 verglichen mit den Werten vor Propranolol-Einnahme. Aus: Brodde et al. [24]

beschrieben worden. Nach plötzlichem Absetzen des Propranolols nahm die β_2-Adrenozeptordichte nur langsam wieder ab und war noch nach 3—5 Tagen signifikant erhöht, obwohl bereits nach 24 Stunden kein Propranolol im Plasma mehr nachweisbar war (Abb. 8). Eine solche „Supersensitivität" von β-Adrenozeptoren nach plötzlichem Absetzen von Propranolol könnte die Ursache für das „Propranolol-Entzugs-Syndrom" sein [28].

Auf der anderen Seite führte Pindolol, ein nicht-selektiver β-Blocker mit ISA (2 × 5 mg/Tag) zu einer signifikanten Abnahme der β_2-Adrenozeptordichte in den Lymphozyten (Abb. 9), in Übereinstimmung mit kürzlich publizierten Ergebnissen von Molinoff und

Aarons [29] und Giudicelli et al. [30]. Nach Absetzen des Pindolols nahm die β_2-Adrenozeptordichte nur sehr langsam wieder zu und war noch nach 4 Tagen signifikant erniedrigt, obwohl bereits nach 36 Stunden kein Pindolol im Plasma mehr nachweisbar war. Es ist gut verständlich, daß unter diesen Bedingungen ein plötzliches Absetzen von Pindolol nicht zu Rebound-Effekten führen sollte, da sich keine „Supersensitivität" der β-Adrenozeptoren entwickeln kann. In der Tat sind Rebound-Effekte nach plötz-

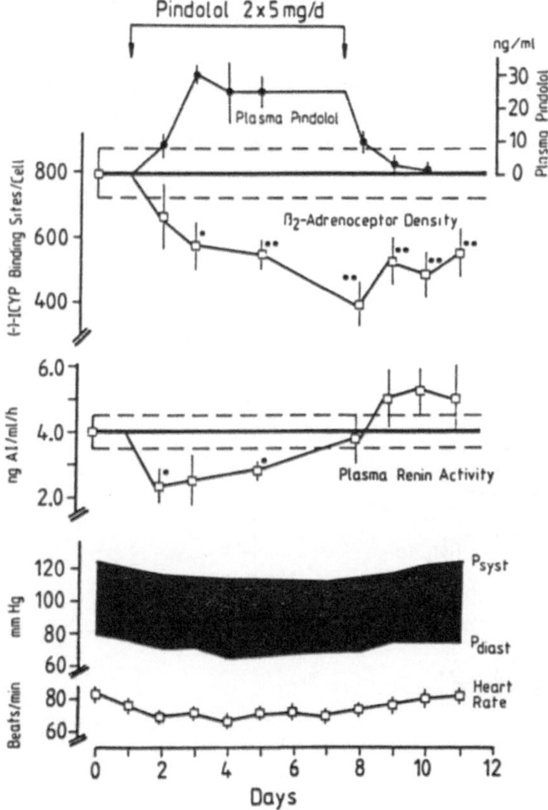

Abb. 9

Einfluß von Pindolol (2 × 5 mg/d) auf β_2-Adrenozeptor-Anzahl, Plasma-Renin-Aktivität, Blutdruck und Herzfrequenz bei 8 gesunden Probanden.
Ordinate: (von oben nach unten): β_2-Adrenozeptor-Anzahl in Lymphozyten — bestimmt durch Scatchard-Analyse [9] der ICYP Bindung — in ICYP Bindungsstellen/Zelle; Plasma-Renin-Aktivität in ng Angiotensin I gebildet/ml/Stunde; Blutdruck in mmHg und Herzfrequenz in Schläge/Min. *rechts:* Plasma-Pindolol-Spiegel in ng/ml.
Abscisse: Versuchstage
Angegeben sind Mittelwerte ± mittlerer Fehler des Mittelwertes. Durchgezogene Linien und gestrichelte Linien: Mittelwerte ± mittlerer Fehler des Mittelwertes vor Pindolol-Einnahme. **) P < 0,01 *) P < 0.05 verglichen mit den Werten vor Pindolol-Einnahme. Aus: Brodde et al. [25]

lichem Absetzen von Pindolol bisher nicht beobachtet worden [31]. Propranolol (3 × 40 mg/Tag) verhinderte die durch Pindolol hervorgerufene Abnahme der lymphozytären β_2-Adrenozeptor-Dichte vollständig (Abb. 10), was dafür spricht, daß für die β-Adrenozeptor reduzierende Wirkung des Pindolols seine ISA verantwortlich ist.

Im Gegensatz zu Pindolol und Propranolol hatte der hochselektive β_1-Blocker Bisoprolol [32] ohne ISA (1 × 10 mg/Tag) keinen Einfluß auf die β_2-Adrenozeptordichte in den Lymphozyten, weder während der Behandlung noch nach Absetzen (Abb. 11). Die Tatsache, daß der β_1-Adrenozeptor Antagonist Bisoprolol ohne ISA — im Gegensatz zu dem nicht-selektiven β-Adrenozeptor Antagonisten Propranolol ohne ISA — die β_2-Adrenozeptoren in den Lymphozyten nicht beeinflußt, spricht sehr dafür, daß Pharmaka-hervorgerufene Veränderungen der lymphozytären β-Adrenozeptoren subtyp-selektiv β_2-Adrenozeptorveränderungen widerspiegeln. Diese Befunde schließen nicht aus, daß Bisoprolol als β-Blocker ohne ISA (wie Propranolol) zu einem Anstieg von β_1-Adrenozeptoren (z.B. im Herzen) führen kann, und somit nach plötzlichem Absetzen Symptome einer β-adrenergen „Supersensitivität" auftreten könnten.

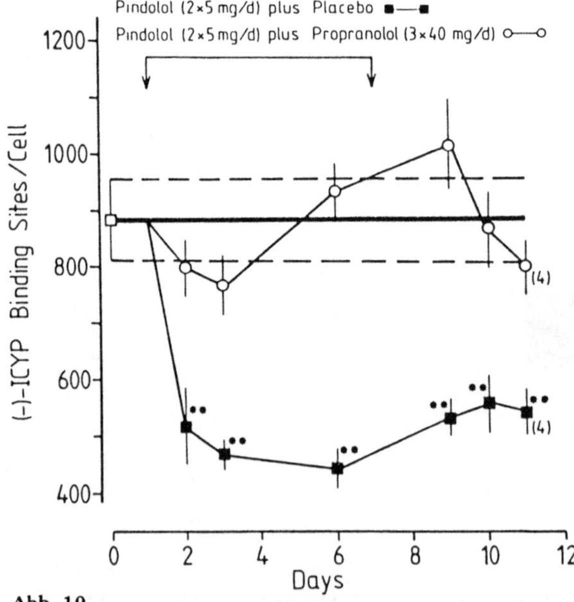

Abb. 10

Einfluß von Pindolol (2 × 5 mg/d) *plus* Placebo (■–■) oder Pindolol (2 × 5 mg/d) *plus* Propranolol (3 × 40 mg/d; ○–○) auf die β_2-Adrenozeptor-Anzahl in Lymphozyten von 8 gesunden Probanden. *Ordinate:* β_2-Adrenozeptor-Anzahl in Lymphozyten — bestimmt durch Scatchard-Analyse [9] der ICYP-Bindung — in ICYP Bindungsstellen/Zelle.
Abscisse: Versuchstage
Angegeben sind Mittelwerte ± mittlerer Fehler des Mittelwertes. Durchgezogene Linien und gestrichelte Linien: Mittelwerte ± mittlerer Fehler des Mittelwertes vor Einnahme der β-Blocker. **) P < 0.01 verglichen mit den Werten vor Einnahme der β-Blocker. Aus: Brodde et al. [25].

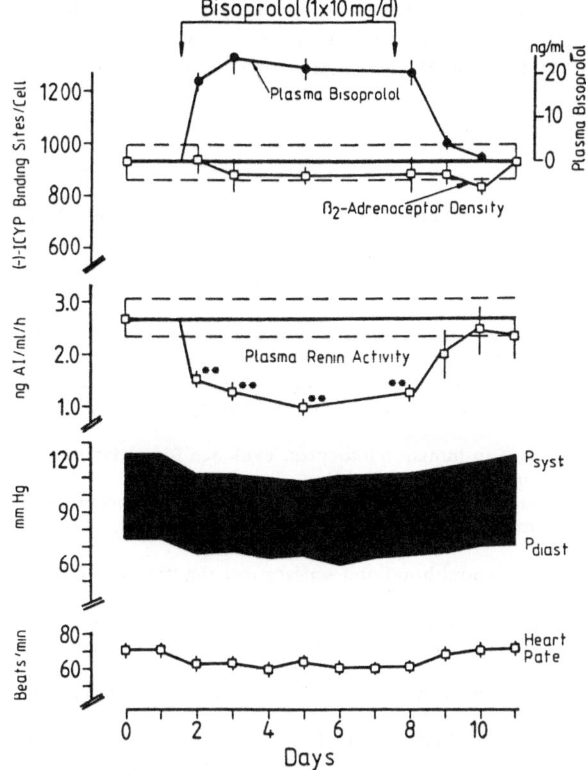

Abb. 11

Einfluß von Bisoprolol (1 × 10 mg/d) auf β₂-Adrenozeptor-Anzahl, Plasma-Renin-Aktivität, Blutdruck und Herzfrequenz von 12 gesunden Probanden.
Ordinate links: (von oben nach unten): β₂-Adrenozeptor-Anzahl in Lymphozyten — bestimmt durch Scatchard-Analyse [9] der ICYP-Bindung — in ICYP Bindungsstellen/Zelle; Plasma-Renin-Aktivität in ng Angiotensin I gebildet/ml/Stunde; Blutdruck in mmHg und Herzfrequenz in Schläge/Min.
rechts: Plasma-Bisoprolol-Spiegel in ng/ml.
Abscisse: Versuchstage
Angegeben sind Mittelwerte ± mittlerer Fehler des Mittelwertes. Durchgezogene Linien und gestrichelte Linien: Mittelwerte ± mittlerer Fehler des Mittelwertes vor Bisoprolol-Einnahme. **) P < 0.01 verglichen mit den Werten vor Bisoprolol-Einnahme. Aus: Brodde et al. [25].

Zusammenfassend zeigen die Befunde der vorliegenden Arbeit, daß die Bestimmung von β₂-Adrenozeptoren in zirkulierenden Lymphozyten eine geeignete Methode ist, um am Menschen Veränderungen in der Funktion von β-Adrenozeptoren zu bestimmen. Da wir kürzlich zeigen konnten, daß Veränderungen in der Anzahl von β-Adrenozeptoren in Lymphozyten signifikant mit Veränderungen in der Anzahl und Ansprechbarkeit von β-Adrenozeptoren im Herzen der gleichen Patienten korrelieren [33], scheinen lymphozytäre β-Adrenozeptor Veränderungen repräsentativ für β-Adrenozeptor Veränderungen in anderen Geweben des Menschen zu sein. Die genaue Kenntnis pathologisch- und pharmakologisch-hervorgerufener Veränderungen in Anzahl und Ansprechbarkeit von β-Adrenozeptoren sollte neuartige, gezielte therapeutische Maßnahmen ermöglichen.

Literatur

[1] *Lefkowitz, R. J.:* Identification and regulation of alpha- and beta-adrenergic receptors. Fed. Proc. 37, 123–129, 1978.

[2] *Hoffman, B. B., Lefkowitz, R. J.:* Radioligand binding studies of adrenergic receptors: new insights into molecular and physiological regulation. Ann. Rev. Pharmacol Toxicol, 20: 581–608, 1980.

[3] *Williams, L. T., Snyderman, R., Lefkowitz, R. J.:* Identification of beta-adrenergic receptors in human lymphocytes by (−)-^{3}H-alprenolol binding. J. Clin. Invest.; 57: 149–155, 1976.

[4] *Brodde, O.-E., Engel, G., Hoyer, D., Bock, K. D., Weber, F.:* The β-adrenergic receptor in human lymphocytes: subclassification by the use of a new radio-ligand, (±)-^{125}iodocyanopindolol. Life Sci.; 29: 2189–2198, 1981.

[5] *Bourne, H. R., Melmon, K. L.:* Adenyl cyclase in human leukocytes: evidence for activation by separate β-adrenergic and prostaglandin receptors. J. Pharmacol Exp. Ther. ; 178: 1–7, 1971.

[6] *Brodde, O.-E., Daul, A. E., O'Hara, N., Khalifa, A.M.:* Properties of α- and β-adrenoceptors in circulating blood cells of patients with essential hypertension. J. Cardiovasc Pharmacol; 7 (Suppl. 6): S. 162–167, 1985.

[7] *Roth, G. S.:* Hormone receptor changes during adulthood and senescence: significance of aging research. Fed. Proc.; 38: 1910–1914, 1979.

[8] *O'Hara, N., Daul, A. E., Fesel, R., Siekmann, U., Brodde, O.-E.:* Different mechanisms underlying reduced β_2-adrenoceptor responsiveness in lymphocytes from neonates and old subjects. Mech Ageing Develop; 31: 115–122, 1985.

[9] *Scatchard, G.:* The attraction of proteins for small molecules and ions. Ann. N. Y. Acad. Sci.; 51: 660–672, 1949.

[10] *Abrass, I. B., Scarpace, P. J.:* Human lymphocyte beta-adrenergic receptors are unaltered with age. J. Gerontol; 36: 298–301, 1981.

[11] *Landmann, R., Bittiger, H., Bühler, F. R.:* High affinity beta-2-adrenergic receptors in mononuclear leucocytes: Similar density in young and old normal subjects. Life Sci.; 29: 1761–1771, 1981.

[12] *Doyle, V., O'Malley, K., Kelly, J. G.:* Human lymphocyte β-adrenoceptor density in relation to age and hypertension. J. Cardiovasc Pharmacol; 4: 738–740, 1982.

[13] *Middeke, M., Remien, J. Holzgreve, H.:* The influence of sex, age, blood pressure and physical stress on β_2-adrenoceptor density of mononuclear cells. J. Hypertens; 2: 261–264, 1984.

[14] *Abrass, I. B., Scarpace, P. J.:* Catalytic unit of adenylate cyclase: reduced activity in aged-human lymphocytes. J. Clin. Endocrinol Metab; 55: 1026–1028, 1982.

[15] *Motulsky, H. J., Insel, P. A.:* Adrenergic receptors in man. Direct identification, physiologic regulation and clinical alterations. N. Engl. J. Med.; 307: 18–28, 1982.

[16] *Davies, A. O., Lefkowitz, R. J.:* Regulation of beta-adrenergic receptors by steroid hormones. Ann. Rev. Physiol; 46: 119–130, 1984.

[17] *Bretz, U., Martin, U., Mazzoni, L., Ney, U. M.:* β-Adrenergic tachyphylaxis in the rat and its reversal and prevention by ketotifen. Eur. J. Pharmacol; 86: 321–328, 1983.

[18] *Brodde, O.-E., Brinkmann, M., Schemuth, R., O'Hara, N., Daul, A.:* Terbutaline-induced desensitization of human lymphocyte β_2-adrenoceptors. Accelerated restoration of β-adrenoceptor responsiveness by prednisone and ketotifen. J. Clin. Invest.; 76: 1096–1101, 1985.

[19] *Stadel, J. M., Strulovici, B., Nambi, P., Lavin, T. N., Briggs, M. M., Caron, M. G., Lefkowitz, R. J.:* Desensitization of the beta-adrenergic receptor of frog erythrocytes: recovery and characterization of the down regulated receptors in sequestered vesicles. J. Biol. Chem.; 258: 3032–3038, 1983.

[20] *Davis, C., Conolly, M. E.:* Tachyphylaxis of beta adrenoceptor agonists in human bronchial smooth muscle: studies *in vitro*. Br. J. Clin. Pharmacol.; 10: 417–423, 1980.

[21] *Lane, D. J.:* A steroid sparing effect of ketotifen in steroiddependent asthmatics. Clin. Allergy; 10: 519–525, 1980.

[22] *Lebeau, B., Gence, B., Bourdain, M., Loria, Y.:* Le ketotifen dans le traitement preventif de l'asthme. Poumon-Coeur; 38: 125−129, 1982.

[23] *Kumagai, A., Tomioka, H., Shida, T., Takahashi, T., Muranaka, M.:* Clinical evaluation of a new orally active anti-anaphylactic compound: ketotifen (HC 20-511) in Japanese adult asthmatics. Schweiz Med. Wschr.; 110: 197−203, 1980.

[24] *Brodde, O.-E., Daul, A., Stuka, N., O'Hara, N., Borchard, U.:* Effects of β-adrenoceptor antagonist administration on β_2-adrenoceptor density in human lymphocytes. The role of the "intrinsic sympathomimetic activity". Naunyn-Schmiedeberg's Arch. Pharmacol.; 328: 417−422, 1985.

[25] *Brodde, O.-E., Schemuth, R., Brinkmann, M., Wang, X. L., Daul, A., Borchard, U.:* β-Adrenoceptor antagonists (non-selective as well as β_1-selective) with partial agonistic activity decrease β_2-adrenoceptor density in human lymphocytes. Evidence for a β_2-agonistic component of the partial agonistic activity. Naunyn-Schmideberg's Arch. Pharmacol.; 333: 130−138, 1986.

[26] *Aarons, R. D., Nies, A. S., Gal, J., Hegstrand, L. R., Molinoff, P. B.:* Elevation of β-adrenergic receptor density in human lymphocytes after propranolol administration. J. Clin. Invest.; 65: 949−957, 1980.

[27] *Wood, A. J. J., Feldman, R., Nadeau, J.:* Physiological regulation of beta-receptors in man. Clin. Exp. Hypertens; A4: 807−817, 1982.

[28] *Prichard, B. N. C., Tomlinson, B., Walden, R. J., Bhattacharjee, P.:* The β-adrenergic blockade withdrawal phenomenon. J. Cardiovasc Pharmacol.; 5 (Suppl. 1): S 56−S 62, 1983.

[29] *Molinoff, P. B., Aarons, R. D.:* Effects or drugs on β-adrenergic receptors on human lymphocytes. J. Cardiovasc Pharmacol; 5 (Suppl. 1): S 63−S 67, 1983.

[30] *Giudicelli, Y., Lacasa, D., Agli, B., Leneveu, A.:* Comparison of changes in the characteristics of β-adrenoceptors and responsiveness of human circulating lymphocytes during chronic and after chronic administration of pindolol and propranolol. Eur. J. Clin. Pharmacol.; 26: 7−12, 1984.

[31] *Szecsi, E., Kohlschütter, S., Schiess, W., Lang, E.:* Abrupt withdrawal of pindolol or metoprolol after chronic therapy. Br. J. Clin. Pharmacol.; 13 (Suppl. 2): 353S−357S, 1982.

[32] *Wang, X. L., Brinkmann, M., Brodde, O.-E.:* Selective labelling of β_1-adrenoceptors in rabbit lung membranes by (−)-^{3}H-bisoprolol. Eur. J. Pharmacol.; 114: 157−165, 1985.

[33] *Brodde, O.-E., Kretsch, R., Ikezono, K., Zerkowski, H.-R., Reidemeister, J. Chr.:* Human β-adrenoceptors: relation of myocardial and lymphocyte β-adrenoceptor density. Science; 231: 1584−1585, 1986.

Sachwortverzeichnis

für deutschsprachige Beiträge

Subject Index

for English contributions